Dialogues between Psychoanalysis and Architecture

Dialogues between Psychoanalysis and Architecture explores the multisensory space of therapy, real or virtual, and how important it is in providing the container for the therapeutic relationship and process.

This book is highly original in bringing psychoanalysis and architecture together and highlighting how both disciplines strive to achieve transformation of our psychic space. It brings together contributions that comprise three parts: the first explores the space of the consulting room through the senses to examine issues such as smell and its link with memory and belonging, hearing out the Other, the psychoanalytic couch, the medical therapy room and the so-called sixth sense; secondly, the book questions how the consulting room can represent or be redesigned to reflect the philosophy that underlies the therapy process, foregrounding an architectural point of view; and thirdly, the book attends to the significance of the consulting room as a virtual space, as it emerged during the pandemic of COVID-19 and beyond.

Architectural, psychotherapeutic and interdisciplinary perspectives allow for an important new dimension on the psychological use of space, and will appeal to psychoanalysts, psychoanalytic and integrative psychotherapists, art therapists, students of psychotherapy, as well as architects and designers.

Christina Moutsou, Ph.D., is a psychoanalytic therapist, social anthropologist and author. She has worked as a lecturer and supervisor in various academic institutions and organisations, and in private practice in London for more than 20 years. Her publications include *Fictional Clinical Narratives in Relational Psychoanalysis* (2018), and her debut novel, *Layers* (2018).

'I cannot recall the last time that I encountered such a truly *original* book. Drawing upon her training in both mental health and, also, anthropology, Dr. Christina Moutsou has curated a deeply compelling collection of essays by talented writers, who transport us on an engaging tour of the consulting room through the senses. I only wish that I had absorbed all of this wisdom decades ago when I rented my very first consulting room! This volume should be required reading for psychoanalytical trainees and practitioners of ever age and shape and size.'

Brett Kahr, *professor; senior fellow at the Tavistock Institute of Medical Psychology, London; visiting professor of psychoanalysis and mental health at Regent's University, London; and honorary director of research, Freud Museum, London*

'How does the physical and sensory space of the consulting room impact on the psychic space that develops within psychoanalysis? And in the wake of the COVID-19 pandemic, how does the use of the virtual therapy room change or facilitate analytic work? Christina Moutsou is to be congratulated on providing us with a wonderfully original and stimulating book that addresses these and other timely questions. With the help of distinguished contributors from the fields of both psychoanalysis and architecture, she has created a fascinating dialogue between disciplines that are too rarely considered together.'

Rosemary Rizq, *Ph.D., CPsychol, AFBPs, FHEA, Professor Emerita of Psychoanalytic Psychotherapy, University of Roehampton, London, UK*

'This book comes as an extraordinary gift to let us reconsider the complex relationships between imagining and creating spaces, the senses, and the process of crafting a psychoanalytic mind. Even in the face of pain and loss, emerging from the bound and the ordered allows us to claim unanticipated freedom in the fragility and vitality of the senses to retrieve the spontaneity of wonder, shift the drivenness of the mind, and achieve growth.'

Emmanouil Manakas, *Ph.D., psychoanalytic psychotherapist, North Hellenic Psychoanalytic Society*

Dialogues between Psychoanalysis and Architecture

The Relational Space of the Consulting Room Through the Senses

Edited by
Christina Moutsou

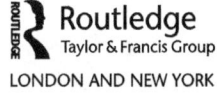

Designed cover image: Photo by Eleni Papaioannou, http://elenipapaioannou

First published 2024
by Routledge
4 Park Square, Milton Park, Abingdon, Oxon OX14 4RN

and by Routledge
605 Third Avenue, New York, NY 10158

Routledge is an imprint of the Taylor & Francis Group, an informa business

© 2024 selection and editorial matter, Christina Moutsou; individual chapters, the contributors

The right of Christina Moutsou to be identified as the author of the editorial material, and of the authors for their individual chapters, has been asserted in accordance with sections 77 and 78 of the Copyright, Designs and Patents Act 1988.

All rights reserved. No part of this book may be reprinted or reproduced or utilised in any form or by any electronic, mechanical, or other means, now known or hereafter invented, including photocopying and recording, or in any information storage or retrieval system, without permission in writing from the publishers.

Trademark notice: Product or corporate names may be trademarks or registered trademarks, and are used only for identification and explanation without intent to infringe.

British Library Cataloguing-in-Publication Data
A catalogue record for this book is available from the British Library

Library of Congress Cataloging-in-Publication Data
Names: Moutsou, Christina, editor.
Title: Dialogues between psychoanalysis and architecture : the relational space of the consulting room through the senses / edited by Christina Moutsou.
Description: Abingdon, Oxon ; New York, NY : Routledge, 2024. |
 Includes bibliographical references and index.
Identifiers: LCCN 2023018825 (print) | LCCN 2023018826 (ebook) |
 ISBN 9781032388007 (hardback) | ISBN 9781032388045 (paperback) |
 ISBN 9781003346845 (ebook)
Subjects: LCSH: Psychotherapists' offices—Design and construction. | Psychiatric consultation—Environmental aspects. | Psychoanalysis and architecture. | Architecture—Psychological aspects.
Classification: LCC RC465.5 .D53 2024 (print) | LCC RC465.5 (ebook) |
 DDC 616.89/17—dc23/eng/20230731
LC record available at https://lccn.loc.gov/2023018825
LC ebook record available at https://lccn.loc.gov/2023018826

ISBN: 978-1-032-38800-7 (hbk)
ISBN: 978-1-032-38804-5 (pbk)
ISBN: 978-1-003-34684-5 (ebk)

DOI: 10.4324/9781003346845

Typeset in Sabon
by Apex CoVantage, LLC

To George, for being there over the years

Contents

Acknowledgements xi
List of contributors xiii

Introduction 1
Christina Moutsou

Part 1: The relational space of the consulting room through the senses 13

1 In the beginning is smell: the sense of belonging and remembering and the impact of its loss in psychotherapy 15
   Christina Moutsou

2 Hearing other voices: the ear as the eye of invisible class discrimination 30
   Anastasios Gaitanidis

3 Touching nostalgia and regret when lying to tell the truth on the couch 39
   Christina Moutsou and Salma Siddique

4 The therapy consulting room in a medical setting as experienced through the senses 55
   Vanessa Pilkington

5 Unfurling Ariadne's thread: psychic connections and the engagement of the 'sixth sense' in the consulting room 68
   Christina Moutsou

Part 2: Dialogues between architecture and psychoanalysis — 81

6 On the architect's couch: elective affinities between architecture and psychoanalysis — 83
Korina Filoxenidou and Katerina Kotzia

7 Dialogues between architecture and psychotherapy: revisiting four consulting rooms — 99
Korina Filoxenidou and Natalia Varfi

Part 3: The online consulting room during the COVID-19 pandemic and beyond — 121

8 The screen therapy room: real flowers in a digital vase — 123
Dora Tsogia

9 Sensual deprivation and therapy during the COVID-19 pandemic — 146
Christina Papachristou

10 Observing and consulting in the digital aquarium: exploring the shifting waterscapes of online therapy — 162
Salma Siddique

Index — 176

Acknowledgements

As described more fully in the introduction, the process of editing this book has been somewhat fragmented and complicated, as I took on the sole editorship while undergoing a challenging health journey during the dark times of the pandemic. I would like to thank all the contributors for accompanying me and inspiring me during what at times felt like an uncertain obstacle course. Each one of them was very significant in the process, and their support at various stages of the long journey of bringing this book together from conception to publication made a real difference.

During the early stages of working on the book, Anastasios Gaitanidis and I ran an experiential weekend workshop for the training student group in the Philadelphia Association on the consulting room, real and virtual. This felt like an extensive session of brainstorming where we were inspired and learnt a lot from the students, and we were able to 'meet' them in their online consulting rooms. Korina Filoxenidou and Katerina Kotzia joined for the conclusion to the weekend workshop and offered an architectural point of view. Some of the comments of the students are included in a few of the chapters in the book anonymously, with their consent at the time. I would like to thank all the students present in that early workshop for their contributions and Jake Osborne, the Chair of the P.A. training committee, for facilitating our access to the student group.

I am particularly grateful to Kate Hawes, the psychoanalysis editor at Routledge for trusting me with all the changes and delays that editing the book required, and for showing faith in me and the project. Georgina Clutterbuck, the editorial assistant at Routledge, has been a discreet, responsive and facilitating presence all along. I am very grateful to Brett Kahr for his generosity to me and his interest in the project. Rachel Milroy and Chryssa Anagnostopoulou-Tsoukis have supported me professionally and personally throughout the process of editing the book and provided listening spaces for me to express my thoughts about the book and, at times, to vent. I would like to thank Eleni Papaioannou for the generous donation of one of her photographs for the front cover. Damien Doorley provided invaluable space, inspiration and listening, which made a difference.

The final stages of editing the book felt somewhat like an exercise in endurance and solitude. George Kapetanios has faithfully stood by me, as always, and provided concrete, practical, but mainly emotional support when it was needed the most. For that, I am enormously grateful and touched.

Contributors

The editor

Dr. Christina Moutsou is a social anthropologist, psychoanalytic psychotherapist and published author of fiction. She obtained her Ph.D. in Social Anthropology on hybrid representations of ethnic identities in Brussels (U. of Cambridge, 1999). She subsequently trained as a psychoanalytic psychotherapist (Philadelphia Association, 2002). She has co-edited three books in anthropology and psychotherapy and has published several papers in academic journals. More recently, she has published her debut novel, *Layers* (Akakia 2018) and a collection of fictional short stories in adolescence and in therapy (Routledge, 2018). Her novel and short stories have been translated into Greek. Christina has held several academic and supervisory positions (visiting lecturer at Birkbeck and Regent's Universities, clinical and research supervisor at N.S.P.C. and Islington Mind). She has been working as a therapist in private practice in London since 2002 (www.space-for-thinking.co.uk). She is a senior member of the Philadelphia Association and the Site for Psychoanalysis. Christina has an interest in the interrelationship between psychoanalysis, fiction and sociocultural context as well as in working with complex trauma in long-term open-ended therapy.

The contributors

Korina Filoxenidou is an architect and educator. She has taught Architectural and Interior Design in private and public institutions in Greece and has led numerous student workshops. Since 2018, she is an assistant professor of Architectural Design at the School of Architecture of the University of Ioannina. Korina is a founding member of K&K Architects studio. The studio deals with the design of small and large-scale works, as well as the curation and design of art and architecture exhibitions. Her research interests revolve around the notion of ephemerality in design and the experiential and interactive nature of ephemeral architecture.

Anastasios Gaitanidis, Ph.D., is the director of Relational Psychoanalytic Therapy Ltd, a relational psychoanalyst, author, theory editor and supervisor. In addition to his clinical work as a psychoanalyst, Anastasios held appointments as a senior lecturer and director of studies, and provided clinical and research supervision to counselling psychologists and psychotherapists at Regent's University London, Metanoia Institute and University of Roehampton. Anastasios is the Theory Editor of the *European Journal of Psychotherapy and Counselling* (E.J.P.C.) and an author who published a substantial body of academic work including journal articles and edited books over the years, with a recent book publication entitled *The Sublime in Everyday Life: Psychoanalytic and Aesthetic Perspectives* (Routledge, 2021).

Katerina Kotzia is an Architect, AUTh. (1997), Master of Arts in Design Studies from Central Saint Martin's College of Art and Design (2000) with a scholarship from the Onassis Foundation. She is an Assistant Professor of Architectural Design at the School of Architecture of the University of Ioannina (2018). Since 2019 she also teaches Exhibition Design and Curation in the Postgraduate Program of the School of Fine Arts of the University of Ioannina. She is a founding member of the K&K Architects (2000–) a practice that specialises in the curation and design of architecture exhibitions.

Christina Papachristou, Ph.D., is a clinical psychologist and psychodynamic psychotherapist and currently Assistant Professor for Clinical Psychology at the Aristotle University of Thessaloniki, Greece. She has worked as a clinician and researcher for more than fifteen years in the Department for Psychosomatic Medicine at the Charité University Hospital in Berlin, Germany where she built up on her interest in the interrelation of psychology and the body with a special interest in the field of organ transplantation.

Vanessa Pilkington, Ph.D., is a chartered psychologist working in the central London area. She worked in the voluntary and N.H.S. sectors for ten years before setting up her independent practice in 2010. She has a wealth of clinical experience working with clients experiencing life, emotional and psychological difficulties. Her interests include the varying ways people experience emotional suffering that may be diagnosed as a psychological and emotional disorder, a topic fully researched in her Ph.D. (City University). She is an ongoing contributor to *The Article* on psychological matters and has also contributed to *The Telegraph*.

Salma Siddique, Ph.D., an Associate Professor of Psychoanalytic Anthropology in Human Development at Connecticut College, USA, Supervisor and Clinical Anthropologist is a curious explorer of the human psyche, fascinated by the intersections of existential philosophy and medical humanities. Through her research, she attempts to delve into the depths of psychoanalysis, psychotherapy and anthropology, seeking to unravel the mysteries of our collective consciousness. Salma's unique approach blends fact with fiction, creating friction that challenges established paradigms and illuminates new perspectives. Her fragmented pieces dance along the margins, blurring the boundaries between imagination and empirical data, defying potential pitfalls and betrayals of categorisation. With each mark, she expands our understanding of the relational other, inviting us to explore uncharted territories within ourselves.

Dora Tsogia, Ph.D., studied at the Aristotle University of Thessaloniki (B.A. in Philosophy, Psychology and Education), at the University of Stirling (M.Sc.) and at the University of Birmingham (Clinical Psychology Doctorate). She has twenty-five years of clinical experience in the U.K. and Greece, both in the public sector and in private practice. She has lived in Athens, Greece since 2004, where she works as a Clinical Psychologist – Psychodynamic Psychotherapist. She has a special interest in psychotherapy of trauma and in issues concerning women's mental health (pregnancy, I.V.F., menopause, etc.). She is also a playwright and has published two books with works for the theatre.

Natalia Varfi is an architect. She graduated from the Department of Architecture, University of Ioannina in 2022. Her research interests revolve around the effects of interior space in human psychology. Her research thesis explored the dynamic of the psychotherapy consulting room space, through a series of questionnaires handed to psychotherapists and students of psychotherapy. Her diploma dissertation was a project-based thesis on four case studies, four consulting rooms, belonging to four therapists in Greece and the U.K.

Introduction

Christina Moutsou

History in dialogue

Psychoanalysis introduced a revolutionary method where personal history was being recorded through dialogue. The history of this project is also inscribed in dialogue. It all started just before it was officially announced that a global pandemic was looming, in December 2019, when a number of friends and colleagues attended the launch of my therapy fictional short stories in Thessaloniki, Greece. The idea took a while to form fully, but it took shape as a co-writing project between Anastasios Gaitanidis and Christina Moutsou on the therapy consulting room in dialogue with two architects, Korina Filoxenidou and Katerina Kotzia, who were conducting qualitative research on the space of the therapy consulting room. Those early days of the project included many extensive conversations between the four of us and brainstorming, partly inspired and partly fuelled by the loss of the actual space for embodied meetings and the collective need to connect virtually during the frightening time of global hospitalisations and deaths while we were all in lockdowns. The concept of examining the space of the consulting room through the senses was an idea that I developed during a difficult moment in the early days of the pandemic (see Chapter 1). It provided a somewhat ironic and nostalgic reference to what had been lost during a time of massive trauma, how we are all rooted in our bodies and in lived and shared experience.

Eventually, a proposal for a co-written book in conversation was submitted to Kate Hawes, the psychoanalysis editor at Routledge, in the summer of 2020 and was gracefully approved in the autumn of the same year. But in the meantime, the pandemic was unfolding alongside life with all its multiple predicaments during such dark times as well as the consolidation of the reality that the consulting room was actually one of the casualties of the pandemic, while the demand for online therapy had hit the roof, and while therapists alongside other keyworkers were on the frontline of a mental health crisis. In our conversations about the book, we often swapped notes about how overwhelmed we felt with clinical and/or academic tasks and, eventually, Anastasios withdrew from the project. After much trepidation and while facing my own difficult journey, I took on the editorship of the book and Anastasios, Korina and Katerina all endeavoured to contribute with chapters. I was now on the lookout for other contributors.

The delay and complications in forming the present project turned out to be meaningful. As the pandemic unfolded further and more contributors emerged along the way, it became clear that this was developing into a project about the embodied and the virtual consulting room through the senses as well as the relational ground of the therapy room as the potential third holding and enveloping the therapeutic dyad. What was being gained and what was being lost in relation to the space of the consulting room during the pandemic? It felt like many threads were emerging and coming together, space for dialogue, history, relationship, space for discomfort, trauma, loss and recovery through resilience.

Psychoanalysis and architecture

I was fortunate to be introduced to the striking parallels between psychoanalysis and architecture well before the conception of this project through conversations with friends. In his book, *The Poetics of Space*, Bachelard describes eloquently how human beings' psychic expression is embedded in the creative use of physical space (Bachelard, 2014). Sperber (2016) draws a parallel between psychoanalysis and architecture in how both disciplines are a creative response to human predicaments through building a relationship, which entails careful listening. Daedalus, she says, the first ever architect, was able to navigate his way out of the labyrinth through building a bridge.

Traditional psychoanalysis' focus though, Sperber (2016) points out, is on loss and mourning through accepting emotional reality, while architecture can appear to put the emphasis on phantasy and creation as an escape from frustration and the suffering of human limitations. Sperber juxtaposes Daedalus with Icarus, who was fixated on his omnipotent wish to construct wings that would get him to fly high, near the sun, which ended in his tragic, mortal crash as opposed to building a bridge through mutual respect in a relationship, which was Daedalus's strategy. Such juxtaposition is also reflected and elaborated on in the architectural chapters in this volume.

In her revisiting of the Jewish Museum in Berlin, an unsettling formulation of space by the renowned architect Daniel Liberkind, which has been designed with the purpose to unsettle the visitor through recreating the effect of the Holocaust on those who had to endure it, Domash (2014), a psychoanalyst who is interested in wider applications of psychoanalysis in the arts, writes a case study of how she personally experienced a visit to the museum. Like in the process of analysis, where dark demons can get stirred up and faced, Domash claims that her sense of being unsettled, nauseated and the vertigo she experienced while in the space of the museum had a therapeutic effect in that it helped her connect her with the history of ancestors, what it felt like to be a Jew of the Holocaust. In his response to Domash's paper, Gerald (2014) points out that not all visitors of the museum agree with Domash's interpretation of the experience. Some found it abusive, as though they were violently and forcefully induced to a cruel and deliberately damaging psychic experience.

This raises the important question of whether psychoanalysis and architecture should be aiming to comfort or to unsettle, or both. Are the psychoanalyst's and architect's attempts to immerse their subject into an inner journey in physical/psychic space a process of potential healing or a process more similar to opening up Pandora's box? And to the degree that it can feel more like the latter, can there be a sound boundary between psychic truth and violation? The approach endorsed in this book primarily by all contributors, though their particular area of expertise or approach may differ significantly, is that the common denominator that may turn a potentially dark journey in physical and psychic space into a process of creative exploration is the relationship built between the subjects participating in the process, i.e., the therapist and the patient or the architect and their client. I had not quite realised before immersing myself into the final stages of editing this book to what degree psychoanalysis and architecture have this in common – a careful and fine-tuning attempt at listening in the context of forming a relationship with the client(s), which entails a profound understanding of the client's psyche before creating a space that can hopefully be transformative and even therapeutic, even though not devoid of the potential to unsettle.

Trauma and resilience

One of the most brilliant and thought-provoking books that I read during the covid crisis was *Freud's Pandemics* by Brett Kahr (2021). In the introduction to the book, aptly entitled *Wouldn't it be better, if we all killed ourselves?* apparently an uttering of Anna Freud when she was cross-examined by the Nazis, Kahr observes that Freud went through several pandemics during his life, not only the historically recorded Spanish Flu pandemic, one of the tragic casualties of which was his daughter Sophie, who left behind her two young children (Kahr, 2021, p. 63), but many other periods of sociopolitical upheaval and extreme trauma, such as World War II and losing his home and becoming a refugee in his eighties while suffering with terminal cancer. Kahr describes his book as a *trauma biography* of Freud's life, as the series of upheavals Freud endured throughout his life left him with a collection of wounds and scars, but also with a remarkable ability to survive and rise above trauma through the creativity of his mind, which constituted a new form of true resilience, psychoanalysis, a method that transformed our cultural and sociopolitical arena and formed the landscape of our understanding of subjectivity in the 20th and 21st century.

Another two recent publications on the psychological impact of the pandemic also explore the pivotal relationship between trauma and resilience in their unique ways. Vos's book, *The psychology of Covid-19* (Vos, 2021) is an exploration of how the risk assessment and the psychology of fear can trigger mental fragility. He writes:

> When I became ill with meningitis-like symptoms in 2006 during an epidemic in an African region where I had been working, the virologist told me that I had three options: 'death, chemotherapy, or a miraculous natural recovery', – I 'chose' the third option.
>
> (2021, pp. 1–2)

In another recent publication, *The Covid Trail* (Brunning & Khaleelee, 2023), a co-edited book on the psychological impact of the pandemic, focussing on recovery through resilience, the editors describe how the COVID trail was a desperate attempt to resist the psychological impact of the first lockdown through discovering an exciting itinerary around London that would also become a point of connection with others who felt equally isolated.

Taking on the editorship of this book during uncertain and unsettling times felt like an act of resilience and a risk. Dufourmantelle (2019) writes:

> Death, we know, is what is risked in us. Holding it imaginarily in our sights is no guarantee that we'll be more living or more loving. If risk is the event of 'not dying', it is beyond choice, a physical engagement at close quarters with the unknown, night, nonknowledge, a wager in the face of what, precisely, remains undecidable. It thus opens the possibility that something unhoped for will happen.
>
> (Dufourmantelle, 2019, p. 7)

It is precisely this possibility of something unhoped for taking place that, I think, has brought this book together through significant risk. A vague seed thrown in conversations between friends just before our world opened up to huge upheaval and darkness took shape slowly and painstakingly into a testimony of the huge importance of the space of the therapy room as a container for a profound embodied relationship. The delay in forming the project meant that the new contributors were able to conceptualise in their chapters the vast changes that the psychotherapy profession is going through with the loss and the re-finding of the consulting room triggered by the collective trauma of the pandemic.

One day in March 2020, we were all asked to work remotely. Little did we know that that day would prove a day of no return for many of the therapy relationships that were being interrupted and disrupted. Some survived the upheaval and were temporarily or permanently transferred online; others never recovered. What could be a more prime example of trauma and of resilience or of resilience through trauma than how we all blindly found our ways to online or telephone work, how we invited our patients to hold on to hope, but also how in some instances the loss of the consulting room and of the embodied relationship were terminal? In the midst of all this, there was a surge for online therapy, new patients finding themselves lost and confounded by what was happening in the world. Some of the chapters in this book speak of these huge changes in psychotherapy, the new and inevitable phase of long-term online work. All of the chapters throw, in some way, their reflective gaze on the impact of the pandemic on the therapy consulting room, real or virtual.

The relational space of the consulting room

What has proven particularly creative about how this project has come together is the various common threads that seemed to exist between us even before conversation took place. For example, two of the initial contributors to the book, Korina Filoxenidou and Anastasios Gaitanidis, were acquainted with Mark Gerald's work, which became a textbook for many of the chapters in this book, before even meeting each other. Gerald, a relational psychoanalyst and a photographer in his book, *Portraits of Psychoanalysts in their Offices* (2020), depicts beautifully how the therapy consulting room is the locus of the therapy relationship with the analyst as the host and the analysand as the guest (Gerald, 2020).

> My approach to imagery, informed by my work as both photographer and psychoanalyst emphasizes appearance and absence. In previous discussions of the spaces and objects in psychoanalytic offices (Gerald, 2011, 2014) I have viewed these rooms as holding environments for the creative potential of psychoanalytic action.

From a relational point of view, the analysand's use of the consulting room is at the centre of the unfolding therapy relationship, as he demonstrates convincingly in his paper, *The stain on the rug*, which tells the story of how a stain of coffee on the rug in his consulting room became a focus of the therapy relationship on more than one occasion (Gerald, 2014). What could have been interpreted as an act of aggression, the accidental spilling of a cup of coffee on his rug by an anxious patient upon the announcement of his forthcoming holiday, seems to present Gerald with a relational opportunity for reflection on attachment and the exposure of the vulnerable self in the therapy relationship.

At the very beginning of the pandemic, I was woken by an anxiety dream. There was a family gathering at a beachside restaurant. The sky had an ominous colour and an alarming sound could be heard from afar. Many of us ran to the waterside where there was sudden warning of imminent danger coming our way, a tsunami perhaps. As my family gathered on the beach, we could all see a foggy scarlet sunset and a little islet just emerging through the fog at the end of the horizon. Was it a symbol of hope or catastrophe? A few days after I had this anxiety dream, my twelve-year-old daughter showed me a painting she had made while feeling bored in her room during lockdown that was identical to the imagery of my dream. A purple/orange seascape and a little rock/island at the end of the horizon. This painting produced at the beginning of the pandemic became the only image all my patients could see during the years of online therapy, as I instantly decided to frame it (with my daughter's permission) and place it on the wall behind me on the right of the camera. Very recently, a patient who has now transferred back to in-person therapy let his gaze fall on the painting. He told me how much it had meant to him during the years of online therapy. His association was with a familiar seascape in Ireland, a place he associates with his roots, which he linked with hope and sorrow. This patient has been through life-threatening illness during the pandemic and is now in the process of recovering from symptoms of trauma.

Being in space through the senses

As Winnicott (1960) has infamously said, there is no baby without a mother, a statement that aptly highlights how rooted we are in the processing of our bodily experience through our senses in the context of a relationship right from the beginning of life. The baby, Winnicott says, can become unintegrated and unhinged through the holding of the mother, who helps her process safely her experience and navigate losing and re-finding herself (Winnicott, 1965). The loss of being rooted in our senses in therapy work, as we largely took it for granted before the pandemic, brought about a tsunami of feelings and posed the urgent question of how we were to process the therapy material under abruptly changing and unpredictable circumstances. Bollas, in his book *Hysteria*, which he understands as a form of maternal disembodiment, also demonstrates how much we are embodied beings who experience the world through all our senses and in relation to one another (Bollas, 1999).

The concept of embodiment has links with French phenomenology and in particular with the work of Merleau-Ponty on intersubjectivity, who focussed on the embodied dance in space that is at the centre of all intimate relationships (Merleau-Ponty, 1945). In her current exhibition at the Munch museum in Oslo entitled *Systems of attachment* (www.munchmuseet.no/en/exhibitions/camille-henrot – mouth-to-mouth/camille-henrot-being-and-becoming-human/), Camille Henrot captures visually the continuity between the intimacy of the maternal container of the baby in intrauterine life and in the oral stage of the physical and emotional symbiosis between mother and baby and all other forms of intimacy through the embodied entanglement of two beings in space, when it is characterised by attunement and affection, without excluding, though, the darker aspects of attachment in its destructive devouring form.

Despite the physical abstinence in the therapy relationship, it became evident during the pandemic, as evocatively demonstrated in the three chapters on the emergence of online therapy work, that the body plays a central role in the mutual processing of the therapy material. How do we process through our senses in online work as opposed to two people sitting in close proximity in a confined space? What is the involvement of the senses required and what is being lost? Can we re-orientate ourselves and become newly integrated through daring unintegration like Winnicott's baby, or is the ultimate risk of the disembodiment of the pandemic some form of permanently disintegrated self, like recent statistics about the rise of mental illness during the pandemic demonstrate?

The space of the consulting room is viewed in this book as the multisensory container of the therapy dyad. In the process of deep and unconscious engagement with one another, which constitutes therapy work, we often do not realise to what degree we intuitively register stimuli through our senses until, as some of the chapters in this book point out, we lose the familiar ground of physicality that contains both parties of the relationship. Of course, the abrupt transfer to online work in March 2020 was a hugely disorientating turn of events that involved significant loss of our sensual engagement as we knew it until then, but also, a possible re-orientation that was both unexpected and potentially delightful, as it was connected with the ability of the human spirit to rise above difficulty. As attachment and neuroscience studies have repeatedly demonstrated, the human brain is particularly flexible and resilient, and in that sense, it is not abrupt separation that is the culprit for permanent damage and trauma, but the inability to heal the damage through reparation and reunion (Gerhardt, 2014). Has anyone noticed the potential for profound disclosure when transferring a therapy session to the phone or how the unexpectedly womblike, safe container of a car can trigger memories previously deeply buried in the unconscious? The consulting room as we knew it, before the pandemic, is undergoing a process of shocking transformation. In online work, we now have two rooms connected through the mediator of a screen or a telephone, rooms that, as some of the contributors point out, would have been concealed from view before.

An outline of the book

In order to mirror the long, but meaningful process that brought all the threads of this book together, it is divided in three parts. The first part, *The consulting room through the senses*, is composed of five chapters focussing on the sense of smell, hearing as a form of biased vision, lying on the couch and its links with touch, the synesthetic impact of the institutional consulting room and sixth sense phenomena in the consulting room. The second part called *Dialogues between architecture and psychoanalysis* is composed of two chapters that highlight the parallels between architecture and psychoanalysis through the discerning sense of taste and the redesigning of four consulting rooms through a process of dialogue and listening. The third part, entitled *The online consulting room during the COVID-19 pandemic and beyond* is composed of three chapters on online therapy during the pandemic and its wider impact and applications.

As an editor, I had to make certain choices with regards to the jargon used in the book as well as the theoretical approaches included. These choices aim to mirror closely the overall relational stance of the book. The relational stance in psychoanalysis (Loewenthal & Samuels, 2014) has a history in being eclectic and sceptical about theory and allowing for a multidisciplinary view of psychotherapy and psychoanalysis. In this respect, though the main theoretical stance in the book is psychoanalytic, there is an emphasis on integrative and eclectic practices with influences from anthropology, the arts and several non-psychoanalytic forms of practicing, such as transactional analysis, body psychotherapy, C.B.T. and existential approaches. In order to allow for such diversity, some chapters are referring to the therapist and patient or client, while others to the analyst and the analysand. The architecture chapters make reference to psychoanalysis as well as to integrative and other modalities of therapy. A number of the chapters include clinical vignettes, which largely follow the principles of composite studies, which is now an established way of fictionalising client discussion in psychotherapy in order to preserve confidentiality (Duffy, 2010). Where detailed case studies have been included in one of the architecture chapters, written permission has been obtained from all the participants.

Following is a brief summary of each of the ten chapters:

Chapter 1, *In the beginning is smell* by Christina Moutsou, focusses on the sense of smell in the consulting room, which is the most under-theorised sense in psychotherapy and other relevant literature. Smell, Moutsou argues, is what the newborn needs to orientate herself to the mother/breast at the beginning of life and is inherently connected with memory, belonging, exclusion as well as intuition. Smell, the intersubjective sense par excellence, is entirely lost as a shared experience in online therapy work.

Chapter 2, *Hearing other voices* by Anastasios Gaitanidis, describes the author's journey to completing this chapter from an overview of the aesthetics of hearing in the consulting room to the realisation that hearing is eclectic and one of the main parameters of exclusion of the Other. Gaitanidis argues that class it the most important denominator of social exclusion and subsequent lack of representation, which is manifested as lack of access to the talking therapies by those who fail to have middle-class sensibilities. He asks the question of how we can begin to hear the voice of the oppressed Other, if our vision is biased through the middle-class affinities of the traditional psychoanalytic consulting room.

In Chapter 3, *Touching nostalgia and regret when lying to tell the truth on the couch*, Salma Siddique and Christina Moutsou review the sociocultural and political history of the couch in psychoanalysis and beyond and offer personal as well as clinical accounts of the use of the couch in therapy work. They highlight how lying down is intricately connected with profound experiences such as being touched and moved in the therapy encounter, early sensory memories, but also the potential for incest, sexual violation and power abuse. The couch, an increasingly controversial piece of furniture in contemporary psychoanalysis, may be in danger of extinction, but maintains crucial links with the sense of touch and its inherent ambiguity within the therapy relationship.

In Chapter 4, *The therapy consulting room in a medical setting as experienced through the senses*, Vanessa Pilkington highlights the difference between the stereotype of the refined therapy consulting room and the realities of working as a therapist in a medical setting. Through focussing on the impact on all the senses during the lived experience of working with clients in the medical therapy consulting room, Pilkington demonstrates convincingly how the therapy relationship is the key factor in how the consulting room can be used as a safe container for the work and how comfort does not have to be the central element in the encounter.

Chapter 5, *Unfurling Ariadne's thread* by Christina Moutsou, examines the place of intuition and the so-called sixth sense in the consulting room through looking at various manifestations of it in the therapy relationship. How to understand psychic phenomena within psychoanalysis has been an issue of controversy, and the terminology used to frame them, such as projective identification and countertransference, as opposed to synchronicity or prophesy, reflects on a historical schism and a lingering discomfort. Moutsou argues that the consulting room can act as the container for the unfurling of the threads that allow for deep psychic connections between the two parties of the therapeutic dyad.

Chapter 6, the first chapter in Part 2, entitled *On the architect's couch* by Korina Filoxenidou and Katerina Kotzia, two architects doing research on the links between psychoanalysis and architecture, is written from an architectural point of view. The authors highlight that *taste* constitutes an entry into the analyst's world by the analysand through the observable and highly personal choices made in the design of the consulting room. They discuss the parallels between architecture and psychoanalysis as processes of deep acquaintance with the Other's world. In the design of the consulting room, one needs to ask the question of how we can move beyond stereotypes that assume that comfort is the main element of the therapy encounter, and conceptualise the unique elements of the psychoanalytic process such as the preservation of history, the dimension of time and its limitations as well as the idea of reconstruction through narrative.

Chapter 7, *Dialogues between architecture and psychotherapy* by Korina Filoxenidou and Natalia Varfi, is based on Varfi's postgraduate qualitative research on the psychotherapy consulting room. The chapter revolves around four case studies of existing consulting rooms that belong to four practitioners. Through an extensive dialogue with the participants about their own individual approach to psychotherapy, how they practise in their consulting rooms and how they would like to better represent their work through the design of the room, the authors suggest a possible redesign of their consulting rooms, which opens up the possibility of a journey of therapeutic change and evolution of their practice for the participants. This is a concrete demonstration through design of the transformative power of dialogue and listening.

In Part 3, Chapter 8, *The screen therapy room* by Dora Tsogia, takes the reader through a journey from in-person to online work during the pandemic, highlighting the complexities of the transfer and the need for thoughtfulness and careful clinical consideration while accepting that a flexible response to the unpredictable changes of the pandemic was necessary. Through a number of fascinating clinical vignettes, Tsogia demonstrates some of the important clinical factors in online work such as a glimpse on the analysand's private space, issues around boundaries and intrusion, the gaze of the therapist when a camera and a screen are the mediators, anxiety and containment in online work, concealment and revelations from both parties, the place of the senses in online work and many others. Tsogia argues that despite the difficulties and potential pitfalls of online work during the pandemic and beyond, digital therapy is effective and proving to be an exercise in resilience.

In Chapter 9, *Sensual deprivation and therapy during the COVID-19 pandemic*, Christina Papachristou focusses her narrative on loss and trauma and the deprivation of the senses through the painful and abrupt loss of the shared embodied space of the consulting room. Papachristou highlights how the therapy relationship is built through the construction of memories that involve the journey to and from the consulting room and the multisensory experiences of sharing the space of the room during the fifty-minute hour. She makes reference to neuroscience research that demonstrates to what extent we are all rooted in our bodies and the physical encounter with one another in space. She links the deprivation in the therapy relationship during the COVID-19 pandemic with the collective trauma and social deprivation we all had to endure. The experience of longing and acknowledging the emotional reality of trauma are at the centre of her argument with regards to online therapy work.

In the final chapter of the book, Chapter 10, *Observing and consulting in the digital aquarium*, Salma Siddique views the online consulting room as a potential transitional object for patients as described in Winnicott's developmental theory. She utilises the metaphor of the digital aquarium in order to highlight how online therapy has the potential to allow either party to be in their natural habitat while engaging with each other, but it can also bring home an experience of deep existential aloneness. Siddique's chapter also throws light onto how future therapy may develop and aptly demonstrates that *tele-therapy* has a long history within psychoanalysis, and that as much as we may resist the change, *digital aquariums of therapy* may be the way forward for many.

References

Bachelard, G. (2014). *The poetics of space*. Penguin.
Bollas, C. (1999). *Hysteria*. Routledge.
Brunning, H., & Khaleelee, O. (2023). *The Covid trail: Psychodynamic explorations*. Phoenix.
Domash, L. (2014). Creating therapeutic "space": How architecture and design can inform psychoanalysis. *Psychoanalytic Perspectives, 11*(2), 94–111.
Duffy, M. (2010). Writing about clients: Developing composite case material and its rationale. *Counselling and Values, 54*(2), 135–153.
Dufourmantelle, A. (2019). *In praise of risk*. Fordham University Press.
Gerald, M. (2011). The psychoanalytic office: Past, present, and future. *Psychoanalytic Psychology, 28*(3), 435–445.
Gerald, M. (2014). The stain on the rug: Commentary on paper by Leanne Domash. *Psychoanalytic Perspectives, 11*, 112–121.
Gerald, M. (2020). *In the shadow of Freud's couch: Portraits of psychoanalysts in their offices*. Routledge.

Gerhardt, S. (2014). *Why love matters: How affection shapes a baby's brain.* Routledge.

Henrot, C. (2023). *Systems of attachment.* Oslo: Munch Museum. https://www.munchmuseet.no/en/exhibitions/archive/2022/camille-henrot-mouth-to-mouth/camille-henrot-being-and-becoming-human/

Kahr, B. (2021). *Freud's pandemics: Surviving global war, Spanish flu, and the Nazis.* Karnac.

Loewenthal, D., & Samuels, A. (Eds.). (2014). *Relational psychotherapy, psychoanalysis and counselling: Appraisals and reappraisals.* Routledge.

Merleau-Ponty, M. (1945). *Phenomenology of perception.* Routledge (Reprinted by Routledge, 2018).

Sperber, E. (2016). The wings of Daedalus: Toward a relational architecture. *The Psychoanalytic Review, 103*(5), 593–617.

Vos, J. (2021). *The psychology of Covid-19.* Sage.

Winnicott, D. W. (1960). The theory of the parent-infant relationship. *International Journal of Psychoanalysis, 41,* 585–595.

Winnicott, D. W. (1965). *The maturational processes and the facilitating environment: Studies in the theory of emotional development.* Routledge.

Part 1

The relational space of the consulting room through the senses

1 In the beginning is smell[1]
The sense of belonging and remembering and the impact of its loss in psychotherapy

Christina Moutsou

In the beginning is smell

During an extensive search in the index of several relevant psychotherapy books, I was not able to locate the keyword 'smell' even once, despite the fact that these were books on the early mother–child relationship and breastfeeding. Yet, smell is the most primary of the senses, how we begin to orientate ourselves, once separated from being inside our mother's body, though perhaps the least talked about. It is the one sense, perhaps alongside touch in the form of skin-to-skin contact, that is the most developed in the newborn baby.

> Olfaction is essential for neonatal behavioral adaptation in many mammals, including humans. Olfactory signals help the newborn baby localize and attach to the nipple at the first sucking bout. Birth and the first hours of life are crucial for olfactory learning. During this period the smell of the mother and that of the newborn interact with each other.
>
> (Bartocci et al., 2000)

Therefore, rooting, the process of the newborn orientating herself towards the mother's breast, is a primary function of smell, the baby finding the mother after birth and the mother letting herself be found. Jacqueline Rose describes how she took naps with her adopted baby daughter, during which she experienced sensations of the baby crawling back into her body, a reverse birth process (Rose, 2018). She describes acutely the physicality and erotic nature of the mother–baby early relationship, which she compares with an affair during which the boundaries of the ego in a bodily sense dissolve, as we accept the other in. She writes: 'I was being turned inside out. This, I suggest, is the chief property of joy, which shatters the carapace of selfhood' (Rose, 2018, p. 200).

Rooting as a concept introduces a relational dynamic in that rather than the baby passively accepting the mother's breast or the mother/breast passively receiving the attack of the baby's insatiable hunger for connection, such as in Melanie Klein's description of the paranoid–schizoid process, there is a *rapprochement*, the baby roots for the mother and the mother roots for the baby. My chapter on the maternal and the erotic in the co-edited book, *The Mother in Psychoanalysis and beyond* (Mayo & Moutsou, 2016, pp. 179–195), begins with a poem on breastfeeding, where smell is a pivotal part of the experience. Here is a short extract:

> **Loss**
>
> . . .
>
> Fragile skin against my skin
> Gently rocking you in my arms
> How I miss your baby smell
> Ice cream texture vanilla and berries
> Jaws that open looking for milk
> Kleinian nonsense breast is only good
>
> (Moutsou, 2016, p. 179).

In her book, *The Shadow of the Second Mother*, Prophecy Coles writes about the history of wet nursing and the obliteration of the working class nursing nanny, who would often exclusively parent a child during their early years. One can deduct from that that a young child's pivotal sensory experiences in early life would be wiped out of memory through the silencing of the widespread practice of hiring a wet nurse among the upper classes. One can only imagine that many of these first sensory experiences would have been olfactory, which also reinforces Freud's argument about smell as the sense closest to the animal instinct that got repressed in humans through evolution (Freud, 1930). It seems to me that the silencing of olfactory stimuli, like the wiping out of the wet nurse as the key parent of young abandoned children, while upper class parents would not deal with hands-on parenting, have a parallel. What is key here is perhaps the silencing of the body as the primary locus of all affectionate bonds of love (Bowlby, 1979).

Smell in clinical practice

The idea of the book in its current form, i.e., the space of the consulting room through the senses, was conceived when I lost my sense of smell through COVID-19. What seemed to be a heavy case of hay fever for a few days was followed by waking up one morning and not being able to smell my first cup of coffee. It is hard to describe the sense of disorientation and disability that I experienced through this unexpected loss. It felt like I could not move freely in space without bumping into things, I could not keep myself safe, to make sure I would not get burned or unwittingly burn the house down without my sense of smell that would normally orientate me. The thought even crossed my mind that life would not be worth living, if that loss of smell turned out to be permanent. I do not intend to overdramatise the experience here, especially as I am aware of the tragic loss of life COVID caused and the significant number of sufferers of long COVID who have learnt to live life through accepting a permanent loss of smell. What I was highly struck by though was how easy it was for bystanders to dismiss loss of smell as not important, while as a society, we do not hesitate to class loss of vision or hearing as serious disability. It seems that there is something about the beginning of life, the primary attunement with a (m)other's body that we may be socio-culturally tempted to dismiss as primitive, to associate it more easily with animal and not with human experience, as Freud suggested (1930). Thankfully, my loss of smell turned out not to be permanent, but the time without it felt unquestionably like a disability, and also, even more strikingly, like a disconnection from life.

While my loss of smell was total, I found it extremely difficult to work clinically as a therapist, even though I felt otherwise well. It was like my ability to tune in to the material in the way I used to before had evaporated. I had become a caricature of a therapist, relying on a toolbox of standard therapy skills in order to orientate myself. In other words, I was no longer able to 'root' for my patients' psyche or to be open to their 'rooting' for me. It was then that I noticed how all the familiar and deeply registered scents of each of my patients and of each therapeutic dyad had also disappeared even before my actual loss of smell through having reverted to online work only during the first abrupt lockdown. I will return to the experience of deprivation of the sense of smell in online work towards the end of this chapter.

The impact my loss of smell had on my ability to practise through attunement, empathy and the ability to register my countertransference was deeply shocking, but also thought provoking. As practitioners, no matter what our personal relationship with theory is, we rely on a theoretical frame through our training in order to conceptualise our work. And yet, what my loss of smell taught me in a much more experiential manner was that the therapy relationship, like all other intimate relationships, is deeply embodied and that it is through the therapist's relationship with the sensory messages within her own body that the connection with a patient is established and deepened. As much as the maternal parallel may have become a cliché in psychoanalytic literature, it seems to me that the therapist does indeed 'root' for the patient, which allows the patient to 'root' for the therapist and to begin the journey of exploration.

Smell and the erotic

The erotic is not to be confused with the sexual, as, like smell, its origins can be found at the beginning of life during that initial attunement between the mother and the baby. During this primarily nonverbal period of life, the task for mother and baby is to communicate through a close bodily connection. Bollas describes eloquently this primary erotic connection of the mother–child dyad in his book, *Hysteria*: 'A mother caresses her infant in countless ways. Whether she nibbles its ears, blows on its stomach, caresses its feet, or tousles its hair, she evokes the child's erotic capability' (Bollas, 2000, p. 44).

For Bollas, hysteria is in fact a cluster of symptoms that could be directly linked with the mother's discomfort or, even, negative reaction to the baby's body and physicality. This links in my mind with the antithesis of the erotic connection through smell, which is the many forms anorexic conditions of purification can take. German Arce Ross describes the scent of anorexia and its link with purification, as one of the strong smells that can infiltrate the consulting room, and which is in antithesis with attunement and the erotic (Ross, 2007, https://m.youtube.com/watch?v=fkwTzUN3JM0&ucbcb=1).

In Stella Acquarone's edited book, *Surviving the early years* (Acquarone, 2016), many examples are given of the crucial importance of body-to-body bonding at the beginning of life, which is also the beginning of the erotic connection with one's own body and that of desired others. A few years ago, I attended a conference on the aftermath of the book's publication. There was a striking presentation on the emotional implications of adoption based on one of the papers in the book, where the presenter stated that in her experience, it is not uncommon for adoptive parents to phone the adoption support agency and report that their babies do not smell right (Raicar et al., 2018). It seems that in some cases of complicated circumstances for establishing parent–child intimacy, eros cannot easily find its way through to olfactory pleasure.

The erotic, a key form of the sublime (Gaitanidis & Curk, 2021), underlies all our important relationships and not only the potentially romantic or sexual ones. As such, it is difficult to conceive of any form of intimacy, where we feel repelled by the other's smell. Sometimes, as I have often experienced in the consulting room with some patients, the scent of the other is not an immediate match. It may, like for those adoptive parents phoning the agency, feel too strong or acrid or lemony or overall not close to the kind of perfume that evokes pleasure. What does this convey about the relationship? Like with other sensory stimuli such as vision, hearing and taste, we can get accustomed and even grow fond of a smell when it becomes familiar. Yet, with smell more so than with any of the other senses, repulsion may prove prohibitive of eros and without eros, a relationship may never be close enough. I also think that there is a primary quality in the sense of smell, precisely because of its pivotal importance at the beginning of life, which makes it less amenable to acquisition. Perhaps, it is not a coincidence that we can conceptualise an 'acquired taste', but not quite an 'acquired smell'.

In one of my short stories, *Mess*, the therapist is guided by the mesmerising effect of the patient's perfume, even though the dialogue is difficult and disjointed and the patient expresses doubt about the therapy and whether she will return. Through the seduction the particular perfume exudes, the therapist experiences in her reverie a cross-cultural journey of discovery, which turns out to be closely matched to the patient's childhood sensual memories. After the end of the session, and while plumping the cushions on the patient's chair, which still exude her perfume, the therapist feels reassured that despite the fragmented dialogue that took place in the session, she will be seeing this patient again. A bond has been established through smell (Moutsou, 2018, pp. 47–51).

Smell and memory

Anthropologists have demonstrated how smell is inherently connected with specific cultural contexts and the social order (Stoller, 1989; Douglas, 1966). We can often distinguish between different cuisines through their distinct use of spices, which evoke olfactory memories from childhood or through lived experience of visiting a place. During my anthropological fieldwork in Brussels on urban representations of ethnic identities through food, I noticed how often spices demarcated whether a particular dish was classed as Greek or Turkish and its equivalent stereotypical representation as 'European' or 'Muslim/Oriental', the latter a category of exoticisation and othering (Moutsou, 1999, pp. 201–204).

I wrote part of this chapter in Antigua, a place I have a strong attachment to, often confirmed through the awakening of my sense of smell while there. It is a series of olfactory memories, which confirm my deep emotional connection with the place. The scent of mosquito repellent and coconut oil on my skin, the freshly grated nutmeg on cocktails, the little clouds of air filled with barbecue aromas, the rising steam of local fish or goat curry, the dust on the roads in the capital of St John's mixed with the salty scent of the ocean nearby, the musky smell of this same dusty ground after a rainfall, the scent of freshly baked pastries and ground coffee beans in the local supermarket.

Smell is inherently connected with memory. There is no other sense that can transport us so quickly to pivotal emotional experiences in our past. It acts as a compass of the psyche, reminding us of the emotional quality of buried, but deeply recorded experiences. In the legendary novel *In search of lost time* by Proust (2019), the narrator recalls a childhood memory through the awakening of the senses that is provoked by smelling and eating a madeleine cake. It is fascinating that the scene of being transported into the narrator's childhood through the olfactory input of the madeleine has become one of the most famous novel scenes in literary history. Perhaps, it has resonated with so many, as an example of how pivotal our sense of smell is in connecting us with our roots in a profound way.

In the consulting room, memory plays a key role in the understanding of the issues faced in the present. Memory can also be terribly biased, which is one of the potential pitfalls of psychoanalytic therapy, constructing fixed narratives of the past, which can become obstacles in living fully in the present. Yet, smell has a unique way of conveying emotional experience in an authentic manner. In other words, our olfactory memories cannot lie as to the quality of our attachments with key childhood figures. Such olfactory memories can also pinpoint accurately where and with whom we have felt at home and/or in what ways home failed to soothe and reassure.

Smell and the excluded other

In her chapter *Beyond the Pale* as part of a co-edited book on homelessness, Gabrielle Brown (2019) writes about the link between bad odour and homelessness, which she says is in fact a prevailing negative stereotype about the homeless, creating distance and consolidating their social exclusion. In truth, she writes, people who are homeless are likely to keep themselves as clean as any of us through access to shelters, where they can shower regularly. Bad odour, she writes, is often connected with experiences of neglect and abuse in childhood, as though the person needs to wordlessly communicate to others their experience of not having learnt to inhabit their body or that their need for being close will intrude and violate the other's space. Of course, bad odour, especially in the small space of the consulting room, can become the locus of the therapist's resentment and disgust or wish to exclude the malodorous Other in order to preserve the space (Brown, 2019). In the prevailing social order, the malodorous can become the ultimate Other.

Unpleasant odour is also often connected with addiction, illness and institutional settings. When Anastasios Gaitanidis and I ran a training weekend in the PA on the five senses in the consulting room, the link between smell and memory came through strongly, especially in relation to the smell of illness and death. One of the trainees recalled working in an addiction centre before the pandemic, and how the strong smell of the fake leather chairs in the room where he saw patients, mixed with the sour smell of alcohol in a particular patient's breath, got imprinted in his memory. Sadly, this patient died later on during the pandemic and so that memory of the smell while in the room with him for what turned out to be the last time was a pivotal experience evoking the emotional reality of this patient's deadly entanglement with the substance. Another trainee recalled the very unpleasant smell of a cancerous ulcer when nursing a family member. She remarked that nobody ever talks about the terrible odour of the dying.

The conversation with the P.A. trainees brought up a memory for me of how the smell of the consulting room when in therapy with a male therapist had changed significantly during a time when my relationship with him had also started deteriorating. What had felt like playful conflict and challenge in our relationship before had shifted to what I experienced as toxic disagreement and a sense of painful rejection, of being the disfavoured one. The unpleasant scent in the room while the relationship was going through a downward spiral was one of the key factors in my decision to terminate the therapy. I had literally begun to find it unbearable to be and breathe in the same room with him. At the time, through virtue of being a trainee in a small psychotherapy organisation, I heard that my then therapist was battling with cancer and was undergoing different kinds of treatment. I think the change in the odour of the room was possibly related to his new health regimes. I still remember vividly my sense of painful guilt for deciding to leave him at a time when he must have felt very vulnerable.

The news of his illness, which had travelled to me, and which I felt unable to share with him, became the elephant in the room between us alongside the unpleasant odour that I was experiencing. At the time, I was in my late twenties and I had spent the best part of a decade since leaving home being worried about my father who was chronically ill and was experiencing regular brushes with death. Having to worry about my therapist as well felt unbearable, but looking back, my inability to be in the room with him in an olfactory way was the most decisive factor. The intrusive presence of a lingering, toxic smell in the room gave me a very clear signal that the relationship was over.

The scent of the consulting room

In his paper, *The stain on the rug* (2014), Mark Gerald reflects on an incident when a patient spilled a cup of coffee on the rug in his consulting room and how that coffee stain became a key factor in more than one therapy relationship as well as an exercise in memory. Gerald is also a photographer, so perhaps not surprisingly he focusses on the visual aesthetics of the stain on the rug. Reading the paper, I wondered what the smell in the room would have been like after the spillage. As much as a cup of steaming coffee exudes a very pleasant aroma, a coffee stain on furniture can have just the opposite effect.

I had once spilled a cup of coffee on my beige couch just before a patient arrived and I felt driven to apologise to her not so much about the visible stain on the couch, which she was thankfully not using, but mainly about the lingering unpleasant smell.

Some of my strongest memories of therapy are about the subtle smell of the consulting room. By now, I have been to several different consulting rooms whether as a patient, supervisee or colleague and smell is always one of the salient confirmations of the embodied experience of therapy, yet the one that is the hardest to think about and acknowledge. Some of my memories of visiting consulting rooms for therapy before are features such as a flower pot with fragrant spring flowers near a window or lavender essential oil in a diffuser, which had taken me some time to locate in the room. I also remember fondly the scent of a cooked casserole lingering in the corridor, as I was walking up the stairs of her house, when my therapist at the time was practising from home. These are, I guess, primarily memories of therapy with a female therapist, when maternal care was one of the qualities I was seeking in the relationship. They are examples of how I had encountered in the room wordlessly and while orientating myself through smell, like newborn babies, the possibility of attunement with anOther (m)Other.

The consulting room does not only smell nice and homely though and it does not always evoke maternal care. It is often a small room with few openings, where receiving one patient after another with a ten-minute break in between, as the traditional practice is, can create a prolonged dysosmia. Since my early days of practising, I have gotten into the habit of opening the window between sessions as well as the door in order to refresh the air in the room, and also in order to attempt to eliminate the traces of each therapeutic dyad. I wonder how widespread this practice is between therapists, and in the typically nonverbal fashion when it comes to the sense of smell, as discussed previously, whether all or at least most therapists open the consulting room's window between sessions, even though none of us is ever taught such a practice in our training.

Like our bodies, each consulting room will have its own particular scent that is unique to the room in question, though influenced by its guests at any one time. Though it is impossible to know what my own consulting room smells like, I can certainly recall how the scent of each consulting room I have been in has left me with a lingering sense of the nature of each therapy or supervision encounter. One important differentiating factor in my mind is whether a consulting room is situated in a house or in an institution or in the crossover between the two. For example, one consulting room I visited for a number of years for supervision was on the top floor of what seemed to be a small block of flats. Though the inside area was airy and fresh in its feel, perhaps slightly infused with the papery scent of a large accumulation of beloved books, the staircase leading to it was dusty and gave out the scent of a neglected, institutional space. Going up and down that staircase always affected my experience, perhaps accentuating the sense of inside versus outside, care versus neglect. It is only through reflecting on the experience now that I am getting in touch for the first time with how central this dual experience of care versus neglect was in that particular encounter. My sense of smell had already inscribed what took me many years to fully verbalise and reflect on, that in that supervisory relationship there was significant confusion about whether care or neglect was the main token.

For me personally, there was a clear preference in being received in a home environment for supervision or for therapy and I think the smell of the consulting room was a key factor in that. The home consulting rooms I can recall smelt 'homely' one way or another, well aired, with lingering pleasant scents of cooked food, some perfume, flowers or essential oils or the subtle scent of artwork and books that lived in the space of the consulting room. The institutional consulting room on the other hand, whether I imagined it or not, smelt of the restrictions imposed by that institution, such as a carpet with an industrial look which triggered sneezing to my allergic constitution during my visits to my first ever therapist or a small room with the standard two chairs at an angle and the coffee table with the box of tissues placed on it and the neutral, office-like scent such a setting may exude. It is also less common in my observation to air a room placed in an institutional setting. It is less easy, though not impossible, for the therapist to create an attunement and identification with the setting of therapy in such an environment. These were the factors that led me to decide to work from home, and yet, I can see that for other therapists or patients the more neutral base of an institutional setting can feel like a safer environment, especially when the sense of a personal space is associated with a fear of boundary crossing and intrusion.

Sensing each other through smell in the dyadic therapy relationship

The erotic attunement at the beginning of life, as outlined by Bollas (2000) and its primary link with physical proximity and therefore smell, also applies to how the connection of the therapeutic dyad gets formed. Even when we do not particularly register a patient's smell, it gets inscribed in memory as a deeply intersubjective experience of being in the room with anOther. As discussed previously, for Bollas, hysteria is a condition resulting from the maternal aversion towards the baby's body. The message that the mother unwittingly gives out is that the baby's body is an object whose orifices need to be cleaned and kept neat, or which needs to be managed without enjoyment and pleasure deriving from the intersubjective nature of the bodily connection. And such dyadic bodily connection is inevitably based on smell, which is the paramount sense that renders the other's body felt and experienced. Interestingly, babies' bodies are also smelly in the traditional sense of the unpleasant odour of bodily excretions. Young babies have very frequent bowel movements, they often vomit milk and it is not uncommon for nappies to leak out urine. Bath time is a traditional time of mother–baby bonding, and yet, what for Bollas turns this cleansing ritual into an experience of erotic connection rather than creating the foundations for body hatred in later life is the pleasure the mother experiences in play and the loving tenderness with which she handles her baby's body.

As I am writing this, Dominique comes to mind.[2] Dominique is an actress who contacted me at the beginning of the pandemic, as she found herself isolated in a house share in London and out of work. She said that other than liking my profile, an important factor in her decision to contact me was my postal address, which was very close to hers. She was hoping we could begin in-person therapy as soon as lockdown rules allowed it. My visual experience of Dominique on screen was strikingly plain. She invariably wore a white blank t-shirt, possibly her sleeping attire, the background wall was also white, she had her hair tied in a ponytail and she rolled cigarettes, which she smoked incessantly. My imagined olfactory experience of her was that of an enclosed space, the air stale and filled with smoke. Dominique came from an Afro-Caribbean background, where, as she explained to me, a lot of emphasis was placed on cleaning her body and making sure there was no intrusion from germs. She had early memories of her mother wiping her clean with strong disinfectant substances. Those memories filled her with anxiety. Other than those daily rituals of cleansing her body, Dominique's mother worked long hours, while she attended early nursery and was often preoccupied with household tasks when she was at home with her. Her father worked even longer hours.

The lockdown affected Dominique badly, in that she only felt alive and desired by others when she was on stage or when she had a strict deadline to prepare for the next show. Enclosed in her small room for hours, she often lost the sense of time as she was surfing the internet and she very frequently forgot to eat and dress. She decided to seek out a therapist when she started experiencing panic attacks that convinced her that she would die alone and that nobody would notice. At the beginning of the work with Dominique, I also experienced anxiety about her deteriorating state of mind, and felt that I needed to see her in person in order to assess her properly.

I eventually met Dominique in person when this was allowed, after four months of online work. She was one of the first patients I met in my consulting room after six months of working online only. The experience is strongly inscribed in my memory. Dominique walked in seeming somewhat anxious and wobbly, but also excited. She was dressed in sporty clothes and dark colours and seemed impeccably clean. This was further confirmed by the scent of fresh soap she gave out as she walked towards the patient's chair. She looked around the room and noticed the essential oil diffuser in my decorative fireplace, a recent acquisition during lockdown. I had in fact bought this when my sense of smell was gone completely, in a desperate attempt to smell something at all while working with patients. She asked me what the scent was and I replied that it was a combination of bergamot, grapefruit and lemongrass. It struck me that the perfumes I had chosen were all clean, citrusy scents reminiscent of warm countries. Later on, she noticed my short wellington boots and the thick socks I was wearing folded over the boots. She said that she really liked this style of shoes. I noted that my boots were still muddy on the side from long walks to the park in rainy weather in an attempt to counteract the effects of lockdown. I silently wondered whether she had also noticed the 'dirt' on my shoes and disapproved.

Dominique no longer appeared plain or unclean like on the screen. She had the body of a gymnast and a performer and someone who was used to being visually exposed to others. It felt like our relationship came alive through this first meeting in my consulting room. Nevertheless, anxiety was very much on the forefront of our interaction as well as the sense that another strict lockdown was looming round the corner. I was also struck by how careful Dominique was about COVID-19 regulations when entering the room. She carefully removed her shoes, bag and coat in the corridor and made sure that she did not touch anything in the room before sanitising her hands. These were of course rules we needed to follow at the time, but her meticulousness made me wonder if she was worried that her body would be a source of fear and anxiety for me like it had been for her mother, unless impeccably clean.

I longed to see Dominique relax into the ritual of coming to therapy, but this was not possible under constantly changing regulations. We discussed how she might find it facilitating to lie on the couch and though she agreed readily, neither of us mentioned it again for a while. I was worried about what an important transition it may be for Dominique to lie down close to me and the effect a future return to online work may have on her, if she took the risk. Indeed, the in-person sessions proved to be intermittent because of changing COVID-19 regulations and eventually the U.K. returned to an even stricter lockdown. Though she always seemed to be understanding and patient with the inconsistency of our meetings, she invariably reported forgetting to eat or sleep at a regular time, when enclosed in her room. She only came alive again when in touch with her housemates or with the boyfriend she had begun dating in the summer. It seemed to me that the embodied in-person sessions as well as activities shared with other people that involved a degree of messiness such as eating together, partying or sleeping with her boyfriend were the only instances where Dominique could feel again that she existed in somebody else's mind.

Online therapy and the total loss of smell

Of course, during the pandemic the sense of smell has not only been lost by some of those suffering from COVID-19; the loss of the sense of smell as a pivotal experience of in-person embodied therapy in the consulting room has also been one of the many casualties. Smell is the one sense entirely lost in online therapy, and yet the importance of this has not been recognised in the growing psychotherapy literature, which seems to suggest that doing therapy primarily online may be the way forward.

My experience of loss of smell through COVID-19 alerted me to the importance of including olfactory stimuli in the therapy relationship. It was striking during that time that I decided to buy an essential oil diffuser for my consulting room. My observation is that I now tend to use it more often on days when I am working primarily online. The conscious choices made by the therapist about the scent of the consulting room, when this is an element the therapist may decide to include, reflects on their conceptualisation of the primal qualities of the therapy encounter. Of course, this will differ from therapist to therapist, not only in terms of their personal taste, but also in terms of how they view the therapy relationship. The oils I chose for therapy work (grapefruit, bergamot and lemongrass) are in my mind clean smelling, aiding reflection, but also evoking a state of leisure (my association here is with a holiday in a warm country). Of course, therapy can be very hard and painful work, but in my view, there is pleasure in it, and without the pleasure of the encounter and of the deep dive into the psyche, the therapy relationship can feel rather sterile.

I have also noticed that many patients bring to their online sessions objects that exude a scent such as a cup of coffee or tea or, quite often, a cigarette that they smoke hastily before ringing the bell. In online therapy, the virtual consulting room is no longer a shared space where the therapy relationship unfolds, but a chosen locus for each of the parties of the therapy dyad with the parameters that make each of them feel comfortable or at home. It is not common to ask patients directly about their everyday relationship with their bodies, especially from an olfactory perspective, and yet, I think this may be a significant factor of where they are in the therapy process. Do they, for example, shower or wear a perfume before their online therapy session? Do they air their room? What if they choose to have the session in their bedroom still wearing their pyjamas? It seems to me that the bodily rituals of online therapy, which can largely remain unspoken, can convey a lot about the issues a patient is working through, but also about their relationship with the therapist.

I have of course asked the same questions in relation to myself. As far as the consulting room is concerned, my rituals have remained unchanged. I continue opening the window between sessions, even when doing online work only, as though the attempt to clear the space for the next session even in the absence of another Body in the room is still pivotal. I also visit the toilet and wash my hands between sessions. These are, I am now realising, rituals of cleansing my body in between sessions in an attempt to symbolically create space for the next patient. I have also dressed and showered daily for work in the same way I did before. Occasionally though, on a busy day, I may steal some time to go out for a run in my break, and I then may have to go straight back into a session without having any time to shower or dress in work clothes fully. Or at times, I have worked online while feeling somewhat under the weather and, on those occasions, I chose comfort over a full work attire. I have noticed that on the few occasions the convenience of online work tempted me to prioritise my own bodily needs over my usual professional embodied self when working therapeutically with patients, I felt somewhat disembodied, as though I needed to resort again to that therapy toolbox for the work. On the other hand, on those occasions, like in the instances when for a session with the camera off, I took the opportunity to sip slowly a warm cup of coffee, which I would not allow myself to do during work on camera, there was also a sense of pleasant regression that could at times benefit the therapy work. It felt like it was more possible in some way to integrate my embodied professional and personal self.

In fact, the freedom to regress may be one of the refreshing and interesting factors in online work for both parties of the therapy dyad. Regression of course is a tricky process, but one that can allow more room for connecting with the unconscious. The patients who choose to have their sessions from their bedrooms, not fully dressed and perhaps not caring about unpleasant body odours in the room, may be regressing to a dysfunctional infantile part of themselves or equally, they may convey that they can take the risk to be seen in their true light. They may also harbour strong fantasies of returning to a place of being taken care of, which would compensate for the gaps of parenting in their childhood. Therefore, online work is potentially opening up the space for the odorous body in its more unhinged form, and for more primitive parts of ourselves that may need to see the light of day in order to be processed.

Smell in the consulting room as an anti-hysterical stance

To conclude, we need to be mindful of the pitfalls of creating a sanitised space in the consulting room, which can have an equally disabling effect on the therapy relationship, like Bollas's account of the effect of the de-eroticisation of the baby's body on the future hysteric (2000). To smell is to be in touch with deep affective experience, which transports us back in memory and to the beginning of life.

I would like to make a case here against neutrality, as when patients get to recognise and respond to the smell of the consulting room, a profound connection has been established. Smell can also register discomfort. We tend to respond in a guarded or aversive way to the odour of purification, as in anorexia, or equally, the intrusiveness of dysosmia such as in cases of self-neglect, illness or addiction. Perhaps, the scent of the consulting room, when it registers for either party of the therapeutic dyad as part of the map of familiarity of long-term therapy, can be evidence of a deep bond.

Notes

1 This subtitle mirrors Christopher Bollas's chapter 'In the beginning is the mother' in his book, *Hysteria* (Bollas, 2000).
2 The case of Dominique here, like most cases and clinical vignettes in other chapters of this book, has been fictionalised following guidelines for the writing of composite case studies (Duffy, 2010).

References

Acquarone, S. (2016). *Surviving the early years: The importance of early intervention with babies at risk*. Routledge.
Bartocci, M., Winberg, J. A. N., Ruggiero, C., Bergqvist, L. L., Serra, G., & Lagercrantz, H. (2000). Activation of olfactory cortex in newborn infants after odor stimulation: A functional near-infrared spectroscopy study. *Pediatric Research*, 48(1), 18–23.
Bollas, C. (2000). *Hysteria*. Routledge.
Bowlby, J. (1979). The Bowlby-Ainsworth attachment theory. *Behavioral and Brain Sciences*, 2(4), 637–638.
Brown, G. (2019). Beyond the pale: Psychotherapy with people who smell. In *Psychoanalytic thinking on the unhoused mind* (pp. 36–55). Routledge.
Coles, P. (2015). *The shadow of the second mother: Nurses and nannies in theories of infant development*. Routledge.
Douglas, M. (1966). *1966: Purity and danger*. Routledge and Kegan Paul.
Duffy, M. (2010). Writing about clients: Developing composite case material and its rationale. *Counselling and Values*, 54(2), 135–153.
Freud, S. (1930). *Civilization and its discontents. The standard edition of the complete psychological works of Sigmund Freud, volume XXI (1927–1931)*. Hogarth Press.

Gaitanidis, A., & Curk, P. (Eds.). (2021). *The sublime in everyday life: Psychoanalytic and aesthetic perspectives*. Routledge.

Gerald, M. (2014). The stain on the rug: Commentary on paper by Leanne Domash. *Psychoanalytic Perspectives, 11*(2), 112–121.

Mayo, R., & Moutsou, C. (Eds.). (2016). *The mother in psychoanalysis and beyond: Matricide and maternal subjectivity*. Taylor & Francis.

Moutsou, C. (1999). *Handling 'food for thought': Greek and Turkish hybrid representations in Brussels* [Doctoral dissertation, University of Cambridge].

Moutsou, C. (2016). The maternal and the erotic: An exploration of the links between maternal and erotic subjectivity. In *The mother in psychoanalysis and beyond* (pp. 199–215). Routledge.

Moutsou, C. (2018). *Fictional clinical narratives in relational psychoanalysis: Stories from adolescence to the consulting room*. Routledge.

Proust, M. (2019). *The prisoner: In search of lost time, volume 5 (Penguin Classics Deluxe edition)* (Vol. 5). Penguin.

Raicar, M., Salkeld, C., & Brenninkmeyer, F. (2018). Adoption and fostering: Facilitating healthy new attachments between infant and adoptive parent. In *Surviving the early years* (pp. 143–163). Routledge.

Rose, J. (2018). *Mothers: An essay on love and cruelty*. Farrar, Straus and Giroux.

Ross, G. A. (2007). Outcomes of smell. *Cliniques Mediterraneennes, 75*(1), 259–275.

Stoller, P. (1989). *The taste of ethnographic things: The senses in anthropology*. University of Pennsylvania Press.

2 Hearing other voices
The ear as the eye of invisible class discrimination

Anastasios Gaitanidis

When I was invited by the editor to contribute a chapter in a book about the five senses in the intersubjective space of the consulting room, I thought that it was a fantastic idea. I was so deprived of the multi-sensorial input afforded by in-person encounters during the COVID-19 pandemic that writing a chapter on how the sense of hearing makes itself present in the therapeutic space would enable me to reflect on this depriving experience and provide a kind of compensation for it. Yet, I found myself time and again not being able to commit to writing this chapter to the extent that I had to recently force myself to think seriously about what I wanted to include in it. This is not a regular aspect of my writing experience: when I feel enthusiastic about a topic, I find myself wanting to write almost immediately about it, to put my nascent thoughts on paper before they are subjected to the vagaries of life and evaporate under the pressure of the relentless assault of everyday worries and preoccupations.

A year into the project and I had only managed to write a couple of pages with my observations and notes regarding the function of hearing in the therapeutic space. Here are a few paragraphs containing my initial thoughts:

> 'I hear you', one might say to convey that one really understands what the other says. Yet, the way this 'hearing' is conducted might register either as an affirmation or a negation of the other's position. Thus, one quickly realises that 'hearing' the other depends not only on what one hears but, most importantly, on how one hears. Hearing thus becomes one of the most complicated senses, generating a constant vacillation from a 'hermeneutics of suspicion' to a 'hermeneutics of trust'.
>
> Hearing is also the most 'distant' of senses: the object that is the source of sound does not need to be present in the vicinity of the subject's domain in order to be heard. For this reason, hearing includes as part of its nature a unique quality: the indication of absence as an anticipation of a potential presence, either benevolent or malevolent, exciting or dangerous, pleasant or shocking. The sound of the patients' footsteps as they approach the consulting room, how they knock at the door or ring the bell are all important

pieces of information for a therapist who often intuits from the quality of these sounds how his/her patients might feel or think.

Moreover, hearing in therapy involves the content as well as the form (the loudness or softness, the pitch and timbre) of a patient's speech, which could be indicative of her/his cognitive and emotional state. Yet, what is often important for psychoanalytic therapy is to keep an ear open for what is not directly said (or remains unspoken) but is implicitly communicated in an intersubjective 'sonic' landscape consisting of beats, rhythms, paces, silences, cacophonies and noises that come from either inside or outside the consulting room and have the potential to interrupt and cause a range of emotions, from amusement to embarrassment to violent ruptures of traumatic anxiety. If 'hearing' is at times privileged over other senses (vision, touch, etc.) in psychoanalysis, it is not the same hearing as the one we employ in everyday life, but a form of listening with a 'third ear', attending to the echoes of the intersubjective 'third' existing in the space between the analyst and the patient.

However, although there was a lot to be said about the 'aesthetic' qualities of the sense of hearing in the consulting room and the importance of creating a space to heed the reverberations of the 'third', I was not satisfied with either the content or style of my writing. While it was academically and aesthetically sound, it appeared contrived and disingenuous, as if I was trying to avoid the embarrassment ensuing from the repercussions of not fulfilling a contractual obligation.

Reading Cynthia Cruz's book

The reasons behind my resistance to, and dissatisfaction with, writing this chapter remained out of reach and invisible until I recently read Cynthia Cruz's brilliant book, *The Melancholia of Class*. Cruz's argument is complex and multifaceted but one of its main premises is that the dominant neoliberal ideology that has established itself since the early 80s with the wholesale adoption of Thatcherite principles of rampant individualism and Reaganomics has convinced us that social classes do not exist, that we all start from an equal, meritocratic basis and resources/opportunities for the creation of wealth and social mobility are available to everyone who is willing to work hard and 'apply themselves'. In this respect, being poor and/or lacking financial, social and cultural capital was the result of one's own 'laziness' and apparent lack of motivation and initiative. In a world where the only acceptable ideological views are those of the affluent middle class, being poor and a member of the working class is no longer either conceivable or possible, as this subject position is not available within the hegemonic neo-liberal discourse. Consequently, members of the working class have been symbolically erased – although they are still alive and materially constrained by their class position, they have been ideologically assassinated. Those who are unable to escape, they are forced to live like zombies, symbolically dead but still carrying on functioning, trapped in a limbo-like space between two deaths. For those who want to survive this violent erasure of their identity, the only way is to abandon their working-class backgrounds and try to assimilate to middle-class values and ideology. However, this assimilation is another form of killing off parts of themselves they left behind, the parts that identified with their lost love object, i.e., their working-class families, friends and neighbourhoods. Thus, they are overwhelmed by feelings of melancholia for what they have left behind and killed off (their lost loved object) since they cannot quite capture or define their loss within the parameters of the dominant discourse. In other words, they are unable to mourn their loss because they cannot locate what is that they have lost either externally or internally. How can they truly leave behind or kill off their working-class origins when the working class is not supposed to symbolically exist in the first place? And how can they return and bury their dead, when there are no corpses to be found – or even if there are corpses, no symbolic funereal rites are allowed to be performed on them by the hegemonic neoliberal discourse?

Now, one might wonder what the relevance of Cruz's argument is for my own resistance to writing this chapter on the sense of hearing in the consulting room. The relevance becomes apparent when one considers the context within which this project was conceived combined with the abandonment of my own working-class background and adoption of middle-class values. I was struck by how excited I was to participate in a project that fundamentally examined the 'aesthetic' quality of the therapeutic encounter – the sensuous aspects of it and their enhancement or curtailment during the time of the pandemic with its concomitant compulsory move to online work – at the expense of its actual, social materiality (financial difficulties, fee structures, accessibility, etc.). It appeared so habitual to me to focus on how our senses function within the new parameters of the therapeutic space (both in-person and online), that is to say, during a precarious time when people (including some of my patients) who mainly belonged to the underprivileged, working class were exposed to potential physical and financial ruin. I, in the comfort and safety of my adopted middle-class environment, protected by the onslaught of the pandemic and having the luxury of maintaining a regular income by working remotely from home, was going to write about how deprived I felt by not being able to experience the full range of hearing afforded by the in-person encounter taking place within the consulting room. It reminded me of what Édouard Louis said about the relation between class and politics:

'For the ruling class, in general, politics is a question of aesthetics: a way of seeing themselves, of seeing the world, of constructing a personality. For us [i.e., the working class] was a matter of life and death' (Louis, 2019, p. 72).

Of course, I am not arguing that the question of the five senses within the intersubjective space of the consulting room is not relevant or should not be asked. I do not want to run the risk of splitting between a 'bourgeois' project concerned with the 'aesthetics' of the therapeutic space and a desired union with the lost working-class Other. I hope that by the end of this chapter I will be able to show how the analytic room could also serve as an important space for hearing the voices of the lost Other once it allows its 'private' container to be infiltrated by the insistent noise of the suffering existing in the 'public sphere'. What I am trying to highlight here is the ease and naturalness with which I asked and attended to this 'aesthetic' question (and others of a similar kind) at a time when I could have also asked other important questions regarding the material conditions, the physical health and the psychological well-being of working-class people. I was surprised and shocked by how unexacting and effortless it was not to think and articulate these questions.

I also felt incredibly guilty for betraying the working-class people I left behind, all those who had no choice but to work and risk (and, in some cases, lose) their lives during the pandemic in order to survive (or help others survive) and who received no material or psychological support. I behaved as if these lives did not matter . . . how was this possible?

Meanwhile, I had experienced an indubitable allegiance to the 'Black Lives Matter' movement instigated by the brutal killing of George Floyd at the hands of Derek Chauvin, a white Minneapolis police officer, as well as to 'Women's Lives Matter' set into motion by the 'Me Too' movement and the horrific rape and murder of Sarah Everard by Wayne Cousens who was serving with the Metropolitan Police (Met) as a police constable and firearms officer. However, I did not register with the same intensity (or, rather, I simultaneously registered and disavowed) the fact that hundreds of thousands of working-class women and men – nurses, ambulance drivers, care workers, train and bus drivers, delivery and garbage disposal workers – were either exposed to deadly dangers or killed every day by a system neither designed nor equipped to protect their lives. And it was not only I that was turning a blind eye to this micro-genocide – it seemed that everyone around me was doing the same too: although there was a clear acknowledgement of the increased danger and rate of mortality within the ranks of the underprivileged and poor, no one seemed to be taking this fact seriously and everyone was treating it as if it was something 'natural' and unavoidable. 'Poor people die – so what's new!' a fellow therapist said to me. 'Nurses, care workers, delivery men – it's their job, right? There is nothing you and I can do about this. Do you expect me to join a 'Working Class Lives Matter' movement? Well, I have news for you: there was a movement like this: it was called Marxism and died a horrible death. Good riddance, I say!' Of course, his callous and insensitive response was the result of his position as a middle-class professional, an established psychoanalyst who completely ignored the suffering of those who were less privileged than him, including the therapists and counsellors who worked hard for the N.H.S. or as volunteers during this period to help contain the *psychological pandemic* that was spreading as fast as the coronavirus one.

Irrespective of this glaring omission, one can also see in his response the explicit signs of the dominant neoliberal ideology that we have all (more or less) come to subscribe to: 'Marxism is dead! The working class is dead! Long live the capitalist market!' The fall of the Berlin Wall signified the failure of Marxism as a political and social programme and the triumph of market ideology with its concomitant rejection of class as a social category. However, what the pandemic (and the recent cost-of-living crisis) made abundantly clear is that class distinctions determine our physical and psychological lives more than ever: it is the working class that has suffered and continues to suffer the most. Of course, one can argue that by focusing on class, one could easily ignore race and gender as important parameters of suffering. Yet, I believe that we should resist this neoliberal line of thinking that is inculcated in us and goes together with its 'divide-and-rule' strategy: by parcelling out suffering into distinct identity categories, neoliberalism has allowed race and gender subject positions to be set against those of class. Of course, one can then conveniently forget how race and gender intersect with class – it is usually Black people and/or women who are amongst the most underprivileged and poorest members of society. To disregard this class distinction and emphasise only race and gender is one of the cleverest ruses that the dominant neoliberal ideology has performed. This does not mean that one should not honour the specificity of suffering derived from discriminations based on race and gender, but this should not be premised on the exclusion of class. These categories need to be thought both together (in their intersection) and apart (in their difference).

Hearing other voices

Now, returning to the question of 'hearing' in the consulting room: in my view, hearing is so central to psychoanalytic work because the function of the analyst is not unlike that of the blind seer, Teiresias, who in Sophocles' (2006) *Oedipus Rex* is able to *see* (and *speak*) the truth of the catastrophic origins of Oedipus's power precisely because he is blind. In a famous exchange between him and Oedipus, when the latter accuses him of lying and conspiring with Creon – his brother-in-law – to usurp his throne, Teiresias replies with the following famous lines: 'To twit me with my blindness – thou hast eyes/Yet see'st not in what misery thou art fallen/Nor where thou dwellest nor with whom for mate'.

The tragedy (and irony) is that Oedipus can only see the outcome of his transgressions when he eventually blinds himself.

In this respect, the analyst, like Teiresias, needs to suspend her/his sight in order to acquire *in*-sight and *fore*-sight. This is because these capacities depend on the development of the analyst's 'imagination' and imagining is not really seeing; it is listening to what is not seen, it is using the analyst's hearing to see the darkness and suffering of what hides behind the visible. The ear thus becomes the eye of the invisible, of what has been concealed, disavowed, and excluded from representation and visibility.

It is the analytic ear, therefore, that could capture the invisible signs of the symbolic assassination of the members of the working class. By listening to the lingering laments of those who have been rendered obsolete by neoliberal ideology, the analyst has the potential to find the words that could give resonance to the cry that is almost inaudible: 'Why have we been killed?'

I am thinking here of one of my patients, a builder in his forties, who had a terrible accident while he was putting up a scaffolding that left him limping but he still needed to work as his disability benefit was not enough to pay the bills. His impotent rage towards the current economic system had gradually found its way into his family life as he began to be verbally and physically abusive towards his wife and children. He hated himself for this – he never thought that he would repeat what his working-class father had done to him when he was young. He came to realise through our work together that both he and his father had suffered so much through years of exploitation and hard manual labour that it was difficult to find anything loving to say to their wives and children. The violence they expressed did not originally belong to them, but it was the unconscious transmission of the violence imposed by the social system that was crushing their bodies and souls.

I am also reminded of another patient, an academic in her late twenties, who suffered from bouts of depression and low mood that she could not understand or explain. During therapy, she realised how she had to abandon her working-class origins in order to fit within the parameters of the middle-class university milieu. Although her 'education' provided her with a ticket out of a 'hard working-class existence' like that of her parents, this assimilation to her new middle-class environment necessitated the unconscious assassination of the parts of herself that identified with (and loved) her working-class family. This produced a form of semi-permanent, low-level depression that could only be mastered and dispelled once she was able to reconnect with her killed-off parts. However, this would not have been possible if I did not bracket off my own preoccupation with creating an air-tight therapeutic container, allowing thus the private sonic landscape of the consulting room to connect with the voices in her working-class background that have been erased by her forced adaptation to what Mark Fisher (2009) calls 'capitalist realism'.

In this sense, analysts need to become aware of their concerns derived from their affiliation with bourgeois sensibilities and values in order to hear and represent the muffled voices of the lifeless and the dispossessed. The impulse behind this hearing involves the active witnessing of the other's suffering, 'of knowing', as Simone Weil (2002) argues,

> that affliction exists, not as a statistic, not as an example from a social category labelled "underprivileged", but as something which happens to a human being, exactly comparable with us, who one day was struck and marked down with a mark that is like no other, by affliction. And to know this it is sufficient – but indispensable – to be able to look at this person with recognition and attention.
>
> (p. 80)

In psychoanalysis, this attention – which is the 'rarest and purest form of generosity' for Simone Weil – is a dynamic that can be described as *thinking with one's ears*. It is a process that allows the stream of *other voices*, the voices of those who have been killed but whose presence still lingers like a ghost, to flow back into the analyst. In achieving the capacity to recognise these silenced voices, the analyst learns to experience this ghostly other as a gift. If so, then, in the flash of a brief moment, a foretaste of redemption can be grasped, and the ghost can be transformed into an ancestor. This is not so much a guarantee but remains a tenuous and surprising possibility.

This is why psychoanalysis remains indispensable to the realisation of Walter Benjamin's 'weak messianism'. According to Benjamin (1992), 'we have been endowed with a weak messianic power to which the past has a claim' (p. 246). This claim addresses us not just from the past but from what will have belonged to it only as an unrealised possibility. For Benjamin, what has never been materialised remains with us as a lingering echo that could gradually transform itself into a secretly unremitting demand. This demand cannot be registered through regular, visible channels of communication; it requires a special attunement, a mode of unconscious responsiveness.

By providing this attunement, analysts could allow the cries of the lifeless and the dead among us to acquire force and expose the brokenness of present life. As analysts, therefore, we are called to overcome our 'refined senses' and 'good tastes' and deconstruct the 'aura' of our private consulting rooms by not treating them as quasi-religious spaces dominated by sacred symbolic imagery and sounds in order to permit the 'unsavoury', 'muted' voices of the members of the working class who have been cruelly persecuted and symbolically erased to *break into* our offices' bourgeois interior. This would involve our attempt to step outside this interior (which, in most cases of psychoanalytic private practice, *screams* class distinction),[1] question our need to immunise ourselves from these 'other' voices coming from the outside world by impressing the dogmatic form of the bourgeois *salon*/living room onto them – something that Benjamin (2002) was keen to identify and criticise as a paradigmatic need of the bourgeoisie in his *Arcades Project* – and participate in political and communal life through multiple activities, including the ample provision of our services to free or low-cost clinics and volunteer organisations.

It is only then that a new 'loudness' can establish itself that can pierce the ears of the neo-liberal elite; and it is only by piercing the ears of this elite that someday the members of the suffering majority could potentially start seeing with their eyes. In the meantime, faced with the sheer volume and rapid succession of advertising, social media and online images, our task as analysts is to help people shut their eyes in order to resist the compulsive hypervisibility of contemporary phantasmagoria and start seeing with their ears the violent nature of their expropriation by capitalist realism.

Note

1 A wonderful example of this 'stepping outside of the interior' is Mark Gerald's project of photographing psychoanalysts in their offices and thus exposing/opening up for the first time this quasi-mystical interior to the public (see Gerald, M. (2020) *In the Shadow of Freud's Couch: Portraits of Psychoanalysts in Their Offices*).

References

Benjamin, W. (1992). Theses on the philosophy of history. In *Illuminations* (H. Zohn, Trans.). Fontana Press.
Benjamin, W. (2002). *The arcades project* (H. Eiland & K. McLaughlin, Trans.). Harvard University Press.
Cruz, C. (2021). *The Melancholia of class: A manifesto for the working class*. Repeater Books.
Fisher, M. (2009). *Capitalist realism*. Zero Books.

Gerald, M. (2020). *In the shadow of Freud's couch: Portraits of psychoanalysts in their offices*. Routledge.
Louis, E. (2019). *Who killed my father?* Vintage.
Sophocles. (2006). *Plays of Sophocles: Oedipus the king; Oedipus at Colonus; Antigone* (F. Storr, Trans.). Project Gutenberg.
Weil, S. (2002). *Gravity and grace*. Routledge.

3 Touching nostalgia and regret when lying to tell the truth on the couch

Christina Moutsou and Salma Siddique

Introduction: lying on the couch[1]

The couch has a rich history in psychoanalysis, but it may evoke multiple associations and feelings (Kravis, 2017; Gerald, 2020). For some, it is like the elephant in the room, a large piece of furniture that certain patients will avoid or never comment on, indicating tactile–emotional violations of early relational trauma, a common element in borderline histories (Van der Kolk, 2015). Others, perhaps with similar relational difficulties and a history of misattuned early attachments, will make a beeline for it before even having the chance to discuss the terms of the work (Shaw, 1996). The couch represents a symbolic terrain for what may evolve in the therapy relationship, even for the patients who do not seem to notice it or who are persistently dissociating from it.

But what about the analyst's cultural and philosophical sensibilities and personal associations with the couch? Mark Gerald, a relational psychanalyst and photographer in his remarkable book, *Portraits of Psychoanalysts in their Offices*, demonstrates through several photographic portraits of psychoanalysts working in various parts of the world not only the organically close relationship between the therapy consulting room and the person of the therapist, but also the centrality of the psychoanalytic couch in many consulting rooms (Gerald, 2020). The couches depicted in Gerald's portraits speak volumes about the identity of the analysts inhabiting the rooms as well as about the socio-cultural context of each analytic setting.

Having talked to colleagues and friends who have undergone analytic training, it is not to be taken for granted that all of them were keen to use the couch or even that they have done so as part of their training analysis. An unacknowledged shift in the sociocultural terrain of analytic therapies overall has been that more therapists are willing to work following their clinical intuition about the dynamics of the relationship in the consulting room rather than be guided by dogma and rigid adherence to orthodoxy. Nevertheless, lying down during analysis can be the closest an analysand can get to receiving physical comfort from their analyst. The material that envelops, the voice that touches and the tears that flow freely can be profound experiences through the sensorial containment of the couch.

DOI: 10.4324/9781003346845-5

The dreams brought to therapy recounted while lying on the couch lend themselves to multiple psychic experiences that are invariably connected to each patient's history and the here and now of the therapy relationship. Associations are with physical touch, which can include its darker sides of sexual violation and incest, regression involving sensory satisfaction and gratification or abstinence from immediate gratification, power imbalances in the therapy relationship, not seeing and its link with trust or lack of it. In all these associations, the body seems to take centre stage in the consulting room through the experience of lying down on the couch. Further, we will explore the felt sense of lying down on the couch and its direct links with touching and being touched.

The couch in the room

Christina

I am writing this in the so-called post-pandemic era, where more of my patients are lying on the couch than ever before. Is this a consequence of the multisensory deprivation of online therapy during repeated lockdowns and COVID-19 outbreaks? Perhaps. There is a broader tendency to observe culture around London and other urban centres, a thirst for in-person meetings, direct contact and interpersonal exchanges that do not entail screens. So, since I have been open to in-person therapy, many of my patients have returned to the consulting room and, even more importantly, to lying down on the couch, a position of potential vulnerability and intimacy.

Interestingly, during the pandemic and while all my patients had reverted to online work, I decided to replace the two therapy chairs and the couch in my consulting room, which had been there for the last twenty years since I began practising, including during one transfer from one consulting room to another. I remember buying those chairs in haste during the move to my first long-term consulting room in West Hampstead. I was newly qualified then and still concerned with keeping to the frame, perhaps overly narrowly. My therapy chairs were neutral, made of a beige leather fabric with wooden armrests. They were comfortable as they were slightly reclining but were rather clinical in accentuating the professional context in which they were being used. My previous couch was a beige day bed with pillows creating a slight recline on the side of the bed closer to the analyst's chair, where a patient would be likely to rest their head with the addition of a blanket by the feet of the bed. Again, the previous arrangement was neutral yet cosy, and the multi-colour cushions provided a warmer accent.

The aesthetic choice I made of new chairs and couch for my consulting room in absentia of real patients visiting it during lockdown seemed to unconsciously throw light on the sense of touch. The new chairs I settled for during the lockdown were blue velvet with a high back and softer armrests. My chosen new couch was a bright purple sofa, which I found to be containing in its shape, as the sides of the sofa provided a comfortable headrest. They opened outwards, giving the sense of an enveloping and safe structure (or at least this is what it felt like to me when trying out the sofa). The couch came complete with three new fur cushions in dark colours. I have witnessed several times when patients, even those who do not lie on the couch, are curious to explore what the cushions feel like to touch.

Was I unconsciously recreating the felt space of the consulting room during an overall abstinence from in-person meetings, preparing the room to receive my patients again after returning to in-person work? During online therapy, several patients commented on the change, as part of the sofa and my therapist's chair is visible on camera.

I am rather unorthodox in how I use the couch in my practice. In a nutshell, I rely on my intuition about the state of the therapy relationship, the history of each patient, and whether lying down according to the previous factors may be appropriate for them in contrast with the classic psychoanalytic position that the couch should be used for 'deeper' analysis and avoided if a patient is working on a less analytic level, such as coming to therapy once a week only.

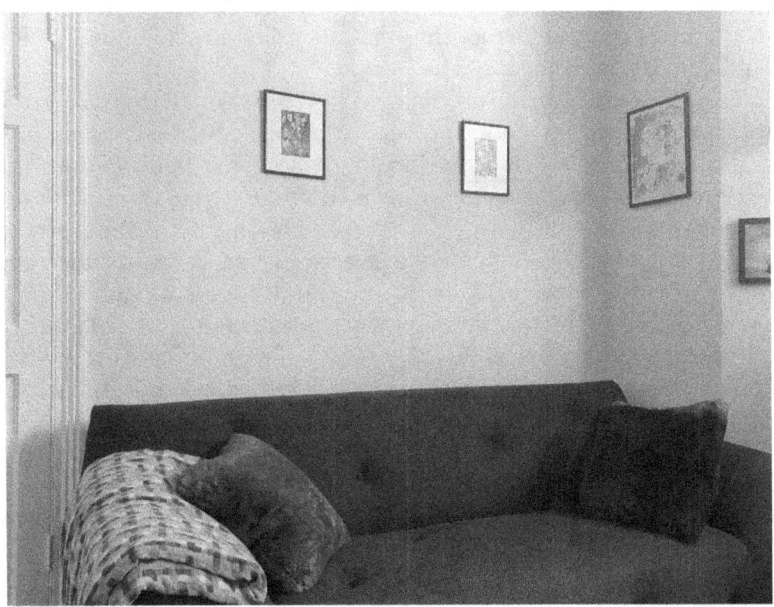

Figure 3.1 My current purple couch

In my experience, patients with a significant history of trauma are less likely to want to lie down (Van der Kolk, 2015), yet may need deep analytic work (Shaw, 1996). Equally, others who may be suffering from feeling a sense of shame often expressed through pervasive self-consciousness may benefit from lying down, even if their discourse may at times seem more superficial. From a relational perspective, the couch and other aspects of the clinical encounter should be part of how two people have been called upon to engage and play with each other. In this sense, my analytic task is more to keep the patient's relationship with the couch in mind (even in its apparent absence) rather than introduce it in the therapy relationship as part of a theoretical framework.

Salma

The couch is a sacred symbol to the therapeutic profession with significance to my life experience. On leaving the psychoanalytic institution and educational centre where I trained, so brutal and systematic was the attack on me in the form of constant questioning of my qualifications and practice that it led to my breakdown and a health crisis that hospitalised me (Siddique, 2018a; Carter, 2022). The couches in my office were donated to a small local charity, as to leave them behind felt like a betrayal. For months later, I dreamt of a couch floating down the turbulent sea before catching alight. My other half often spoke about the goodness of fire and how it is a purifying force that burns away old spirits and bad experiences before welcoming in the new spirits or honouring the fallen heroes (Siddique, 2018b; Siddique & Dominguez, 2021).

The couch in my therapy room is very special to me. It sits in my large therapy room in my house surrounded by bookshelves and paintings and an aquarium. There are Indian rugs on the floor. During the uncertainty of the pandemic, clients who ventured into their in-person sessions perched on the edge of the couch similar to those people who speak of their remoteness experienced like sitting on the edge of the world or an island. Clients spoke of the couch as embodying a shared quality; it became the 'container' for human potential, as they witnessed both themselves and other ways of meaning-making of societal and personal working through social and psychic retreats, which often continues as transgenerational trauma.

I inherited my preloved knoll drop-arm fading brown to a sepia three-seater calf-leather couch from my Italian analyst of several years after Britain chose to leave the European Union (Brexit). He was unhappy with the decision and had decided to return to Europe, if Article 50 was evoked. On 29 March 2017, the fate was sealed and the two-year countdown to the U.K. formally leaving the E.U. began (an

Touching nostalgia and regret when lying to tell the truth

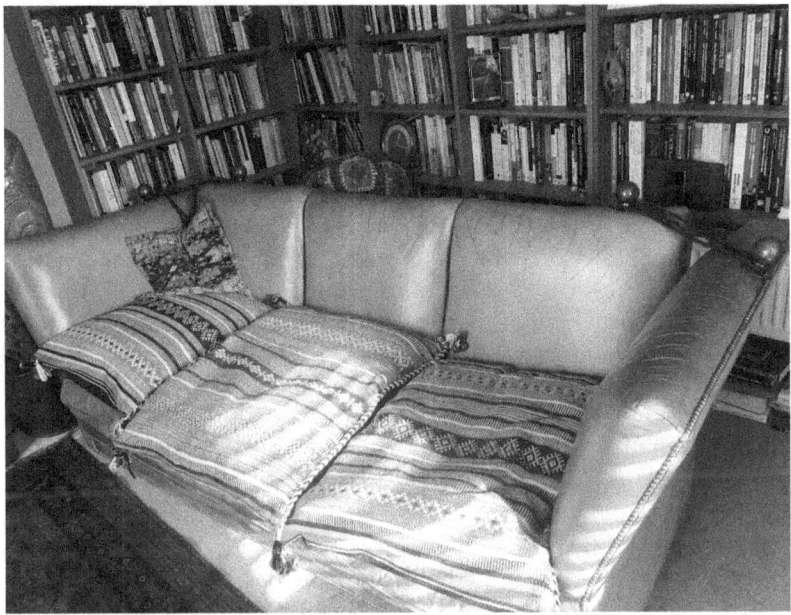

Figure 3.2 The gift of my Italian analyst

act branded by the leavers as 'Brexit'). My analyst prepared to close his practice and leave. In our following session, he announced his intention to leave Scotland within the following year. During the session, I repeatedly asked if the decision was final. I received my answer with a single nod, which felt like our countdown had begun.

He asked me if I wanted a memento of our time together. I looked around in the stark empty room with two armchairs and a couch next to a small wooden side table with a set of coasters on a stand. I reached over and picked out a single mother-of-pearl coaster. Laughter filled the vast space and echoed from my analyst, who sat cross-legged in an armchair. Looking up and shaking his head, he said, instead, he wanted to give me the gift of the couch. Since then, many of my analysands coming into my consulting room or through an online platform often commented that my analyst's couch looked like something out of the Freud Museum in London. The United Kingdom was expected to leave the European Union at 11 pm on 29 March 2019. However, the House of Commons issued a further Brexit extension to 31 January 2020. This became, for me, a liminal transition period. The couch from my Italian analyst had become a threshold between me and the Brexit cultural production, addressing issues of boundaries and difference, the relational perspectives of belonging and not-belonging.

The history of the psychoanalytic couch

The phrase 'sofa' originates from the Arabic word 'suffah' to mean a 'bench', which can be found in 2000 B.C. in Egypt by pharaohs and the affluent classes. However, the Romans started to enjoy all of the sofa's benefits and preferred benches resembling contemporary chaise longues during meals and socialising. As the collapse of the Roman Empire in the 5th century marked the start of the Dark Ages, social life and the sofa were replaced by a bench or stool for the next 1,000 years. Towards the close of the 16th century house development changed and needed to ensure weatherproof living across Europe. A similar revolution occurred with the relationship between carpenters and upholsterers. The sofa became a central aesthetic piece along with the fireplace. From the emerging elegance of Chippendale designs in the mid-1800s, the sofa became the occasional day-bed where one could lie during the day; this signalled the rise of practical designs with cheaper textiles. The sofa became commonplace in households across classes (Warner, 2011).

In his visually captivating book, *The History of the Couch*, Kravis (2017) demonstrates the erotic as well as the medicalised and disempowering potential of the couch well before it was introduced by Freud as the central piece of furniture in psychoanalytic work. In Ancient Greece, the supine position was often associated with nudity and eroticism, a position revisited in the art of renaissance with all its adoring as well as potentially objectifying gaze on the female body. Yet, the predecessor of Freud's use of the couch in psychoanalysis was his neurological studies on hysteria, especially his medical apprenticeship in Paris under Professor Charcot, where hysteria was treated sometimes through hypnosis (Breuer & Freud, 1995). The medicalisation of the female body saw female distress, in the form of the so-called hysterical symptoms, as a narrative of condemnation of female sexuality.

The ultimate challenge of therapy on the couch is to resist the intrusion, leading to remembering. The memories return as flashbacks – moments of the same mind. The couch mediates the consistency of temporality and shapes the space between bodies. Like with Winnicott's baby that cannot exist without a mother, where there is an analyst, there is usually a couch. Always the couch is in the middle of the action regardless of its apparent use by each therapeutic dyad. The patients lying on the couch consent to create a disinhibiting path for free association. When Freud began to use the chaise longue, the patient (most often female) rose from the supine position leaving behind memories and dreams and creating moments of history that marked the beginning of our understanding of human subjectivity. The question remains, given the ambiguity of the history of the psychoanalytic couch, what stories get formed on the couch nowadays and how the blending between fiction and reality that is at the core of the psychoanalytic process through narrative formation may well become a creative integration of 'lying' and profound 'truth-telling'.

What is the impact of the therapist's relationship and free associations with the couch on their ability to use it for therapeutic work? Personal accounts

Salma

The gripping of the arm of the couch and the embracing of a cushion has long been the choreography between two strangers meeting, the witnessing of a possible hope of rekindling. As a therapist, I have witnessed many *rituals* and memorials of meditating, communicating symbolically, bargaining, ultimately touching thoughts and emotions acting as a transition to new inner states and re-claimed social statuses (Nixon, 2005).

Throughout my life, I have been surrounded by couches more like the Indian *Charpai* or remnants of the French day bed whose religion was that of the luxury furniture, seating, and the simplicity of the bed's transforming space between night and day, aesthetic and ambience spaces. Couches came with wooden, silver or brass trimmed legs, embedded with bolsters in a multiplicity of bright colours. As immigrants, the car, television or couch were the first items prominent in the photographs sent back to families left behind in India and Pakistan, considered symbols of luxury. In Pakistan, the couch's simplest forms, swings, were constructed with a wooden board suspended from a tree. More elaborate versions for couples were made from silver or brass and decorated with trimmings, bolsters and gaddas (mattresses).

To have more than one couch is considered a symbol of luxury in certain Indian and Pakistani cultural contexts. Growing up in the U.K. and summering in Pakistan, there was always a women's and men's space with couches in each. Often I have felt that the use of the English couch has been influenced by the Hindi words referring to 'four legs', and the divan in our family home in Birmingham was a more upmarket version of the charpai. It symbolised the seating area of critical, professional and noble guests. However, the charpai was the comfort of the working class used for sleeping or seating multiple people at family celebrations and cultural gatherings (Sanadi et al., 2021).

The couch has also been a place of expansive innovation for me as a child growing up on the couches of my father's mistresses that gave rise to experiences that later became animated narratives of headless figures and distorted bodies making for hybrid myths that followed me around. Ever since, from one consulting room to the next, whether reclining or sitting on a couch, I experience memories that blend together dreamlike existential imagery of (un)comfortable and (un)nerving depictions with the possibility of frustration and disillusionment. What can be experienced and processed horizontally on the couch can be similar to remembering, repeating and working through (Freud, 2001b). As a dual-trained analyst and anthropologist, the couch becomes the site for unfolding mytho-psychological fieldwork.

My earliest memory is that of Sunday afternoons lying back and stretching out, eyes looking straight up at a white ceiling on which hangs the pride of the family, an Italian Murano chandelier my father found in a hardware shop held together by sixty-five glass petals of transparent crystal, smooth outside in a nickel metal frame. The manufacturer recommended light bulb allocation was about eight, to my memory. It was always a significant bone of contention, where silence fell faster than the football kicked by me or my siblings into the light fitting.

Starting therapy from the liminality of adolescence, the couch was an object for illuminating stories of the natural and imagined landscapes across which I travelled many times before finding a way through everyday unhappiness. From the age of four to five, I could imagine sitting or lying on the couch of my father's friend whom he would go to see on Saturday afternoons to listen to music and play chess or backgammon, but never cards because that was gaming for my father. Now when I lie on the couch after all these years, I can recall and experience bodily sensations in my somatic memory of those times left lying on the couch.

On the first occasion in therapy at the age of fifteen, my analyst's open arm gesture directed me to the couch. I glanced at the Eames lounge chair and an ottoman, then I looked at the analyst and then back at the Eames chair; reading the analyst's mind, I took the couch. The couch will give a comfortable distance from his gaze, hence my agreement to see a psychoanalytic therapist. 'They speak and look less'; this process, emphasising reducing or removing eye contact, and its attendant nonverbal communication, may facilitate or hinder free association. The analyst's Naẓar (Shaw, 2021) stands for, in Urdu, the Islamic, what I grew up with, controlling gaze. The senses and, in particular, the 'eye' can be considered as the analytical entanglements between 'seeing' and 'reflecting' which are informed by Islamic and Judeo–Christian understandings of everyday presentation.

The sharing of minds informs the gaze of two strangers who meet at the same time each week in the same place. The psychological process enabled through the gaze enacts the story through language to recognise the relationship(s) to the subjectivity of others; only then do we reveal ourselves. But what can be revealed without the direct gaze? In the myth of the Ring of Gyges (Bloom & Kirsch, 1968), Gyges, the shepherd, received a ring with the power to make him invisible and anonymous. The act of invisibility allows him to seduce the queen, kill the king and become the ruler. Plato (Bloom & Kirsch, 1968) argues that in the narrative of the Ring of Gyges invisibility and anonymity are significant in relationships. Therefore, the in-person and online therapy practice offer different challenges to the psychoanalytical approach. Who is looking at us if we don't look at each other from a seated position? In a recent facilitation of psychoanalytical skills, trainee practitioners spoke about the anonymity of the internet being similar, yet different from when the analysand is out of the gaze of the analyst.

Conversations with a friend reminded me of a childhood experience of visiting with my father his female friend and being placed or invited to sit on the couch and to be lost amongst the cushions or in the books I was reading, which helped me lose track of time and space. The western brain and the eastern mind's reconsideration of psychoanalysis and its informing dominant notions of the sensory were far from universal; sensory phenomena of effect, feelings, desires and bodily sensations of the encounter elucidate inner worlds and intercultural life. I recalled these childhood memories, as I was leaning back on the couch of my recent analyst, sinking into the heavy Moroccan Berber kilim-long pillows. Since then, I have wondered how different shapes and sizes of bodies respond to the containment of the couch. With each session, 'swimming' amongst the long pillows of free association, our body behaves as if it is swimming amongst racing thoughts and anxiety. Diving into a swimming pool is like diving into a therapy session, naturally sinking our body, slowing down the rate of breathing, and keeping near the surface to tread water. I have preferred the couch as a space, a container from which to imagine being held 'in place' amongst the vibrant colours, shapes of fabrics and ornaments, the tessellated ocean of possibilities curated as metaphors of subjectivity grounded in the gaze of the (m)Other. Dialogue, gesture, touch and movement are ways of conceptualising experiences as overlapping cultures that affect this process, focusing on how removing eye contact and its attendant nonverbal communication may facilitate or hinder free association.

Christina

My first encounter with Freud's couch was in adolescence when reading his translated work in Greek and fantasising that one day I would find my way to an analyst's couch and be able to unfold the dark corridors of my mind. That day took a good decade to come about. In my first therapy experience, I scanned the room upon entering to locate the couch, but the room was tiny, and there was none. This was a rather institutional, cosy room at the Cambridge University Counselling Service. The impetus of the institution was to move fast, process difficulties and get on with life, mainly with academic achievement and excellence. This had also been my impetus before entering that room. Therapy was denied to me in adolescence by my parents, who feared I would be facing up to too much darkness, and now, once again, the university agenda was to only scratch the surface. Thankfully, my therapist was analytical and experienced and understood my need for in-depth work. My first therapy couch was self-made in that tiny loft room, where I sat curled up in a foetal ball on the floor cushion surrounded by soft fabric. It was then that I had my first experience of losing my sense of external time and the drive to achieve within fifty minutes of the sensory envelopment of my self-made floor couch. I was almost entirely immersed in the corridors of my mind, and everything else had to pause for a while.

My second experience with the couch was confirmed in what began as a training analysis. I lay flat in that bed, my male therapist beside me, out of sight. I remember the move from the chair to the actual couch and how much I had anticipated it. One of the reasons was that I thought I would feel less self-conscious, less body conscious and scrutinised by his gaze. However, when I started lying down, my therapist's gaze felt even more intrusive in the absence of eye contact and played havoc with my fantasy. I imagined him staring at my cleavage or my exposed hips in their vulnerable position of openness. In fact, sometimes, I would wear revealing clothes to test the theory that his gaze was intrusive and sexualised. My fears were not reassured. The couch I had fantasised about, where I would associate freely and travel in multisensory memory fields, was not yet forthcoming.

My second actual couch emerged when I terminated that first training analysis. I knew it was the kind of couch I had been looking for since the time of turmoil in adolescence when I had first encountered Freud and had fantasised that psychoanalysis would eventually drive me out of the dark labyrinth. The scent in the room travelled me back to early times in my childhood when I would lay my feet on my mother's lap, and she would massage them while I glazed in front of the T.V., to the chamomile tea she would offer me at night as a baby and at times of sickness as well, to feeling cocooned just before falling asleep in my bed when the fragrance of the bedsheets cried out maternal containment. I leaned towards the warm radiator near the couch and was transported to the soothing heat of my childhood, to well-insulated rooms where any draft or dampness would be guarded against. It was a deep wish to be safe in my body that I was touching for the first time. That couch was fertile in what it produced in my life, motherhood and babies that could feed from my body, just like I did on my analyst's couch. Gratification stories always come to an end one way or another. My analyst's couch became much less comfortable as I grew professionally. Like in the myth of Persephone, where the dark horse of sexuality brings about a violent separation between mother and daughter, I was bound to gallop away from that couch onto dark territory.

Some clinical vignettes[2]

Christina

When Ellen first lay on the couch, she transformed into a two-dimensional paper doll, literally vanishing in the natural curves of the three-seater. I felt anxious to get a visual sense of an outline of her body in its three dimensions, but at times, it felt like she had sank deep within the sofa's fabric. Her voice, loud and anxious, fast speaking with no time to draw a breath, contrasted the frail body. When my anxiety became too much to bear, I expressed concern about a particular medication she was taking that was likely to reduce her weight further. She jumped up and yelled at me that she was not there for me to tell her about my anxiety. She lay down again as though exhausted by the fight. She stayed silent for a while. She was there to be contained within my body, the only nourishment she would accept.

His voice was smooth and musical, and the position suited him. He could talk elaborately about his relationship with his wife, his boarding school years and how the past played into the present. I could sense the little boy who pretended to be sick so he could spend some secret time with Mummy at home, get her all to himself like a cake eaten secretly out of a cupboard. I felt moved to tears, which often rolled freely down my cheeks, as I was unseen, and I could tell he loved lying there and losing himself in speaking freely. I remarked once that it was interesting that he never cried, as so much he talked about was deeply emotive. He said the boys who cried at school were the ones who would get abused by the schoolmaster. Instead, all the tears came to me; at least I felt safe letting them flow.

Mary made a beeline for the couch from her first ever session, my consent about how to use this piece of furniture in my room was never quite requested. She sat up in the lotus position facing me head on. I told her hesitantly about how the couch is traditionally used in psychoanalysis and she laughed out loud. She could never imagine lying out of eye contact, she told me! Mary's mother had anger outbursts when she was little. Mary would receive her blows unexpectedly. She had no recollection of what she had ever done to provoke them. She had one memory of running away from home in fear to avoid the beating. Years into the therapy, Mary decided to lie down. Now, it was hip and leg stretches she attempted in the supine position. When I interpreted this as her desire as well as her fear of intimacy, Mary jumped up. She could not tell what it was that frightened her, but she looked like she had just received a blow. This would happen every time she tried to lie down, at a certain point during the session upon hearing my voice, she would sit up abruptly in a fright. After a while, she stopped trying all together.

Salma

I suggested the couch during therapy to one of my clients who was finding it difficult to make and/or retain eye contact. I have worked with Jai, a twenty-one-year-old male, seeing him for at least six months. The reason for the referral was an inability to meet a girl and start a relationship. Jai entered the room and went straight to the couch and lay down at an awkward angle, concertinaed on the length of the couch, facing the back of the couch and tucking his legs under him, exposing the soles of his white trainers. I asked Jai if he was comfortable; he said he didn't know if he wanted to lie or sit on the couch, but he wanted to tell me something and didn't want me to look at him. I replied, well, all I can see from this angle is the blob of designer sports gear crumpled and a pair of white trainer soles, one stacked on the other precariously perched. At that moment he lifted his head and propped his shoulder to turn and look at me. I smiled, I'm still here, and he smiled and dropped his head back onto the cushion.

He slowly emerged from his head buried in the cushion against the back of the couch. I was reminded of an ostrich unfurling its head and neck and presenting surprise and disbelief. I can now think about what I need to know about the client's reflexive position on his experience regarding our ability to engage with both the analytic relationship and the therapist. The activity on this couch is about resistance, free association, transference and the immovable couch. Suddenly the right arm and right leg encircled the air, pointed to the ceiling and then dropped to the ground, and the movement brought the rest of the body into a sitting position. Jai verbalised the first thing that came to mind. 'Don't you think Brexit is bad shit for people like us?' I instantly utter 'Us?' and he comes out with, 'You know? Me and you, us?' I say nothing and just nod as a form of resignation; a moment passes as Jai looks at the fish globe aquarium in the room. I, too, look into the aquarium and see the school of different fish swimming around and think about the hostility and violence met by refugees, asylum seekers and migrants during and after the referendum campaign(s); my own therapist at the time informed me after our seven-year relationship that he had decided that he was returning after having lived in the U.K. for twenty-five years to his home in mainland Europe because of the nature of hostile encounters he had experienced walking home after a social engagement. My therapist spoke about the uncertainty and insecurity he experienced about a sense of identity and belonging. Brexit for those Othered by the process of 'Othering' led to unsettling. Now seven years later, Jai, too, spoke about being called a 'Paki' and told to 'go home to where you come from'. Neither of the men is Pakistani. Narratives of these men are rendered as moments of 'unbelonging' and disruption to social bonding and identity is 'undone'.

Emerging themes

In the process of co-writing this chapter, several themes emerged about what working with and lying on the couch meant for either of us. Some of these themes can be seen as potentially concerning (or even dangerous). They may be viewed as unsettling and uncomfortable, as they touch on the ambiguity of the supine position on the couch and throw light on the multiple layers of meaning of this over-cathected piece of furniture within psychoanalysis as well as on its shadow aspects.

The history of the couch in psychoanalysis has links with its beginnings, which was through the exploration of female sexuality and incest in the Viennese society of the early twentieth century (Breuer & Freud, 1995). Lying down is a position strongly associated with sexual intimacy and/or sexual violation. In the context of parental transference, it can be associated with incest or incestuous fantasies. We tend to close our eyes during intimate physical encounters such as kissing to exclude vision and accentuate our sense of touch.

In the condition of visual deprivation generated by the position of lying down while the analyst is out of sight in the traditional psychoanalytic encounter, the analysand's sense of touch is accentuated just like in other intimate encounters, where visual deprivation becomes a vehicle for enlivening feeling through skin contact. This is the realm of the erotic that encourages an unravelling of the senses through accepting vulnerability as the only authentic condition in all human encounters. Yet, in the traditional analytic position, one party, the analysand, renders themselves vulnerable through surrendering to the gaze of the analyst, whose vision can no longer be met by the analysand's gaze. In other words, in the classical analytic encounter, one of the two parties is required to close their eyes for the kiss that is experienced (in the best circumstances) through the envelopment of the couch (the couching analyst), while the other party's gaze remains unobstructed and unchecked. Where does the gaze of the analyst fall? How is one being seen?

Another aspect of the experience of lying down on the couch for the analysand is connected with evoking regression, as Freud originally intended in his treatment of the so-called hysterical patients during his early work with Breuer, and the multisensory gratification that comes with it. If the analysand is willing and keen to invite regressive states of mind through letting go and allowing oneself to be in the hands of someone else, lying down can be a profound experience of being in touch with one's inner child, innocence and vulnerability through free association and the oral gratification that comes with speaking freely. Freud identified the phenomenon of the 'evenly hovering attention' (being met by an 'open and welcoming mind') where the couch promotes and elicits sensations in the here and now through reverie and the openness of the safely couched body of the analysand. Such experiences have also been described evocatively by Winnicott (Winnicott, 1958), who defined true sanity as the ability to allow for unintegrated states, which require the belief that the mother/analyst will hold the regressed analysand in mind, which will eventually allow for re-integration.

For analysands who struggle to trust the analyst to hold their unintegrated self in a state of regression though (who are likely to be closer to the majority of patients having analytic therapy outside the context of classical psychoanalysis, where it would potentially be claimed that such patients are not suitable for analysis), power dynamics in the therapy relationship may be a central issue that gets introduced in the therapeutic dialogue. Some analysands who strongly oppose the couch point out the incongruence and inequality in the therapy relationship when one part is horizontal, and the other is sitting over them. Can they ever trust their therapist not to abuse their power? The history of the couch in psychoanalysis renders it a symbol of the analyst's status. As such, analysts' personal relationship and associations with the couch are central in how they will choose to place it in the consulting room or even whether they will choose to have a couch at all. It is now becoming common place for rented consulting rooms in London not to have a couch or to include it in the form of a three-seater sofa, which seems to conceal and disavow the original use of the couch within psychoanalysis as a symbol of the analysand's willingness to put themselves in a position of utter vulnerability through truth telling. Sadly, such a position seems to be primarily viewed nowadays as a symbol of the analyst's power and status, which even curated Freud's original Couch as a site of pilgrimage, 'a sacred relic of psychoanalysis' (Nixon, 2005, p. 43).

Conclusion

Is the couch an endangered species in analytical work, and if so, shall we take care to avoid its extinction?

The analysand's positionality of experience in the analysis is their ability to engage with both the analytic relationship and the analyst through conceptualising resistance, free association and transference. Moving away from the analytical couch presence in the consulting room could be seen as a juxtaposition of the comforting, but disruptive of interaction, space of lying down with the relational inviting of dialogue on interaction chairs. Such transition can be literally and symbolically both a barrier and a bridge between transference through eye contact and the unravelling of desire through free association. The therapeutic setting that entails the psychoanalytic couch as a highly cathected piece of furniture where lying and profound truth telling can take place needs to be acknowledged as a historically significant setting before we can safely consider the effect of surrendering this space to the relational chairs of the more mainstream nowadays face-to-face approach.

At times, it is a bleak forecast for the analytical, aka Freudian Couch, and we need to celebrate its long history. We all need to learn how this piece of furniture has raised awareness about the actual conditions that captured our imagination and freed us from aspects of our human suffering throughout the 20th and 21st centuries.

Notes

1 This makes reference to Irvin Yalom's legendary novel *Lying on the Couch* (1997) where the double meaning of the word 'lying' is a central part of the novel's plot.
2 All clinical vignettes in this chapter, just like in other chapters of this book, follow the principles of creating a 'composite case study' (Duffy, 2010).

References

Bloom, A., & Kirsch, A. (1968). *The Republic of Plato* (Vol. 2). Basic Books.
Breuer, J., & Freud, S. (1995). Studies on hysteria. In J. Strachey (Ed.), *The standard edition of the complete psychological works of Sigmund Freud* (Vol. 2, xxxii, pp. 1–335). Hogarth Press (Original work published 1895).
Carter, C. R. (2022). Gaslighting: ALS, anti-Blackness, and medicine. *Feminist Anthropology, 3*(2), 235–245.
Duffy, M. (2010). Writing about clients: Developing composite case material and its rationale. *Counselling and Values, 54*(2), 135–153.
Freud, S. (2001a). The dynamics of transference. In J. Strachey (Ed. & Trans.), *The standard edition of the complete psychological works of Sigmund Freud* (Vol. 12, pp. 99–108). Vintage (Original work published 1912).
Freud, S. (2001b). Remembering, repeating and working-through (Further recommendations on the technique of psycho-analysis II). In J. Strachey (Ed. & Trans.), *The standard edition of the complete psychological works of Sigmund Freud* (Vol. 12, pp. 145–156). Vintage (Original work published 1914).
Freud, S. (2001c). On beginning the treatment (Further recommendations on the technique of psychoanalysis I). In J. Strachey (Ed. & Trans.), *The standard edition of the complete psychological works of Sigmund Freud* (Vol. 12, pp. 123–146). Vintage (Original work published 1913).

Gerald, M. (2020). *In the shadow of Freud's couch: Portraits of psychoanalysts in their offices*. Routledge.

Kravis, N. (2017). *On the couch: A repressed history of the analytic couch from Plato to Freud*. MIT Press.

Nixon, M. (2005). *On the couch*. October, 113, 39–76. Retrieved June 5, 2022, from www.jstor.org/stable/3397653

Sanadi, F. H., Ummah, M. H., & Abdullah, A. (2021). Aqidah of Muslim Sufisme according to the Al-Quran: An analysis. *AL-QIYAM International Social Science and Humanities Journal*, 4(1), 88–97.

Shaw, R. (1996). Towards integrating the body in psychotherapy. *Changes: An International Journal of Psychology and Psychotherapy*, 14(2), 117–120.

Shaw, W. M. (2021). Naẓar, subjectivity, and "the Gaze". In *Naẓar: Vision, belief, and perception in Islamic cultures* (pp. 33–60). Brill.

Siddique, S. (2018a). *Impact of workplace bullying on group cohesion using emotional exhaustion as mediator and neuroticism as moderator* [Doctoral dissertation].

Siddique, S. (2018b). Grace notes XXIV: Mobbing during a time of scarcity. *The Transactional Analyst*, 8(1), 41.

Siddique, S., & Dominguez, V. R. (2021). Anthropology in the consulting room: An interview with Salma Siddique by Virginia R. Dominguez. *American Anthropologist*, 123(1), 179–183.

Van der Kolk, B. (2015). *The body keeps the score: Brain, mind, and body in the healing of trauma*. Penguin Books.

Warner, M. (2011). Freud's couch: A case history. *Raritan*, 31(2), 146–163.

Winnicott. (1958). The capacity to be alone. In *The maturational processes and the facilitating environment*. Karnac Books.

Yalom, I. D. (1997). *Lying on the couch: A novel*. Basic Books.

4 The therapy consulting room in a medical setting as experienced through the senses

Vanessa Pilkington

Introduction

I am a counselling psychologist and work with a variety of clients who are experiencing various manifestations of emotional distress. Their feelings, experiences and problems may be diagnosed as depression, anxiety, stress, trauma and adjustment to name but a few. Ultimately, whatever suffering and adverse life experiences they may report, my role is to help them to gain a deeper understanding of their distress, its triggers and maintaining factors thereby enabling them to manage and overcome it.

As an integrative counselling psychologist, I combine elements of various therapeutic approaches in my work. Cognitive–behavioural, psychodynamic, solution-focused, person-centred and compassion-based therapeutic approaches may all be brought into play. I work in a large and busy central London Medical Centre alongside a team of consultants from different medical disciplines. My clients come to me through different referral paths, through word of mouth, referrals from psychiatrists, general practitioners, other fellow consultants, medical insurance companies as well as from the medical centre in which I work.

I work in a room in a medical setting that is typical of the G.P.'s consulting room. A first impression; bright lighting, walls painted in uniform white, a hardedge desk, a black chunky computer, a heavy printer, wires, an office high-backed wheeled chair and white mini aluminium blinds, limiting the natural light from the small windows that look out onto urban concrete buildings. A blue hospital privacy blind rests just behind the blue examination couch. There is a stark white sink, above which lies a hand washing dispenser and antibacterial gel. The heavy wooden door is shut. There is a discreet alarm close to my chair. The medical setting room often features jagged points and has an office-like feel, a feel commonly associated with tough emotions.

I have attempted to soften this rather severe clinical atmosphere with some fresh flowers and a colourful framed picture. A box of tissues sits on the desk. My coat sits on the back of the door. My bag rests on the examination couch, sometimes with neutral contents spilling out, a magazine, a phone, and maybe some hand cream. My softening attempts notwithstanding, this environment is the antithesis of the soft furnished room one usually associates with the traditional therapy room: comfy sofas, warm lamps, the pretty tissue box, the soft rugs and walls painted in warm colours that draw attention to things pleasant and relaxing rather than to the patient's symptoms and concerns. Perhaps these traditional consulting rooms fuel a diversion or distraction from the content of the therapy session. The traditional therapist's room with its chosen symbolic artefacts often reflects the therapist's taste, which may be deeply personal.

Positive distraction of a slightly different kind is perhaps most obvious in children's hospitals where colours, cartoons and child-friendly images abound, representing an attempt to offset and neutralize any nervous anticipation the child may feel before appointments. An attempt to divert patient attention is here, but the patient is diverted by institutional rather than personal distractions.

In support of the idea that the surrounding space can influence patient/client experience in a therapeutic or medical setting, a study conducted by Andrade and Delvin (2017) suggested that the greater the number of favourable design features in a hospital environment, the lower the patient stress levels. Positive distraction, where one is distracted from a stressor by thinking about or engaging in activities, or perhaps visual distractions, that induce positive emotion, has been shown to lower pain and stress levels in hospital patients. A standard comfy and welcoming therapy space fosters and even facilitates the therapeutic process.

A study conducted by Nasar and Devlin (2011) suggests that the soft environment of the therapeutic space is beneficial to the client's impression of the psychotherapist's office. The more typical therapy room might have comfy armchairs, large windows, soft lamps and perhaps some warm wallpaper as adhered to earlier on. One assumes it would put us at ease and perhaps make us feel at home and relaxed, akin to being in a comfortable living room where we may talk freely and openly with our feet up to a friend or family member. This atmosphere and associated introduction of relaxed feelings may facilitate therapeutic engagement, encouraging a sense of ease, aiding comfort to the disclosing of feelings and thoughts in response to questions. Such an environment is kinder to the sharing of feelings in contrast to the displaying of physical symptoms in the doctor's surgery.

In the medical centre where I work, adults attending for psychological therapy may be comforted by the coffee and tea machine, with its offering of an array of beverages often in patterned colourful boxes. Patient-friendly staff, hot drinks and a welcome reception create institutional comforts, an inviting atmosphere, where people feel acknowledged and looked after. Hospitality puts most clients at ease and makes them feel safe and gets things off to a good start.

Gone, sadly, are the days when magazines and newspapers would lie on tables in front of chairs. Patients would almost regret the practitioner arriving on time, as they sat back with a cappuccino and a magazine or newspaper. The COVID-19 pandemic seems to have wiped this out with the new requirement that nothing be touched by more than one patient.

The light is bright in clinical rooms. This can be an aid in clinical examination and intervention. The cool white light of an L.E.D. bulb is thought to be similar to sunlight. Studies have documented the beneficial effects of such light on reducing depression, decreasing fatigue, and improving alertness. It is thought that cool white L.E.D. bulb light can create the same effect. This is why it is used. It is worth noting that seasonal depression is sometimes treated with bright lamp therapy and that bright light can therefore be associated with mood enhancement. There is a small window in the medical consulting room. Like sunlight, windows and natural daylight have also been shown to increase work satisfaction.

However, the bright light can also arouse a heightened degree of self-consciousness in both therapist and client, perhaps leaving them feeling exposed. This may be especially true for someone who is trying to disclose their inner self and feelings. When talking intimately with someone it can therefore be more beneficial to have softer lighting. Many feelings arise in the room for both client and therapist, and one may not want to feel put 'under the spotlight'.

There is a dimmer on the switch that I often turn right down. Most clients prefer this and feel they can talk more freely. There are, however, occasions when people prefer to have it switched on, usually on more cloudy days. I recall one occasion when the lights were switched off. Having turned them off in the morning when the natural light was strong, the light faded as the day went by. Having been in the room all day, I must have adjusted to it and not noticed the light decline. Only when my client commented 'It is a bit dark in here, can we turn the lights up?' did I notice how the light had lost me over time. Perhaps the bright cool light gives something to those who like it and even request it.

The more traditional therapy room often has a round wall clock ticking away reminding clients of the time and how they may prefer to use it. It tends to sit on a wall visible to both therapist and client. In the room in which I work, a clock sits above the door and during the therapy session only I can see it. Occasionally, there are some clients who turn their heads to look at it, but on the whole, they appear to have no interest in the time.

I introduced a small clock of my own and placed it on the shelf just behind my chair in order to satisfy those who think of the time, how they wish to use it and how much of the session they may have left. Curiously, the majority of my clients never mentioned the lack of clock before this. Maybe this reflects some client ambivalence about the awareness of session time. It seems that some of them like to leave time behind at the door, and it is my job as the psychologist to monitor the time assisting a sense of therapeutic containment in the session. The addition of the clock allows clients who prefer not to surrender control of time to someone else to keep an eye on the time themselves.

In her stories on human compassion and cruelty, Dr Adshead, a forensic psychiatrist and psychotherapist who worked in the N.H.S. within secure hospitals, reflects on her different experiences in private consulting rooms and hospital ones. She refers to the private consulting room as 'a pleasant spot, warm and light' (Adshead & Holmes, 2021, p. 309). She elaborates to say: 'There are no alarms, soft furnishings, the walls are not painted a uniform dirty white and above all there are no locks and no alarms'.

She notes how much she likes it compared to the more institutional hospital or even prison setting. Here, in a similar fashion she conveys her different perception and experience of being in these two opposing settings.

Effects of the medical setting on the client

The medical setting does not offer the comfortable coffee table, plants and plush armchair environment described earlier. But might the harder industrial background encountered in fact lend to the warmth and comfort of the sympathetic and undivided attention of the counselling psychologist?

Could the therapeutic communication be magnified by the contrast? Might the therapist's warm and engaging manner provide a relief to the harsh and clinical backdrop? Might they have to work harder as the client is less likely to just sink into a comfy armchair possibly basking in the immediate and soft setting? As the environment may not put the client at ease immediately, the counselling psychologist may have to compensate instantly in a positive way to counteract this.

The therapeutic relationship is profoundly influential and has repeatedly been found to be the best predictor of therapy outcome. A large study conducted by De Angelis (2019) demonstrated that a good relationship is essential to connect with, remain in and get the most from psychological therapy. Perhaps the relationship is utilised more productively when one is less inclined to get off to a quiet, comfortable start. De Angelis (2019), when reflecting on dialogues between architecture and psychoanalysis, criticised 'comfort' as the main design quality of the consulting room suggesting that comfort and softness have become a stereotypical representation of the therapy consulting room. This chapter argues that it may not in fact be a prerequisite to the success of therapy after all.

Conversely, the medical setting may put the client at ease. People mostly associate medical settings with a feeling of reassurance and safety. One tends to associate a medical centre with an environment of care, where people enter unwell and hopefully and probably leave feeling better. The sight of nurses, suited doctors and occasional medical appliances being wheeled around reinforces this sense of hospital care. Does the hospital environment reduce anxiety and stress for those attending psychological therapy too? Do such elements and amenities reduce stress via perceptions of social support, control and safety?

There is flexibility in the room furnishing and environment however. The examination couch provides alternate use and opportunity. Occasionally, I choose to sit on the examination couch without the office table between me and the client, and it brings a different feel, closer to the sofa and armchair feel, thus removing the more authoritative professional stance. At times this can have a positive effect on certain clients, a greater feeling of relaxation and equality.

I had a client who asked one day if she could lie on the examination couch, thereby hinting at a more Freudian type of therapy session. I asked her why this appealed to her, and she said that there were things she would like to say, without face-to-face direct eye contact. In the traditional form of psychoanalysis, the patient would lie on a couch and not make eye contact with the therapist, encouraging free association where the client may disclose without experiencing negative emotions such as shame or anxiety. This however also precludes a nonverbal response from the therapist that may be of value.

Accommodating this on my part reflects an attempt at flexibility in the providing of psychological counselling in a medical setting.

Conversely, another client's experience of the examination couch was different. Some clients present what is known as hospital anxiety. These individuals feel panicked and anxious when in hospital surroundings. One man disclosed his fear around visiting his mother in hospital. Even the sight of clinical items he referred to as 'scary instruments' raised his anxiety. I asked him how he felt looking around our room. The examination couch he said reminded him of having blood tests. On this occasion, it was helpful for us to be in this environment for the reason that it aroused the very feelings the client was struggling with, thereby enabling us to reflect on them and tackle them directly in the present moment.

The foregoing examples demonstrate how diverse and complex the interaction between client and the therapy room can be.

Sounds

In a busy medical centre, there is not the usual silence one might expect in the classic therapy and counselling setting. The old traditional style of psychodynamic therapy and even counselling today will often incorporate the sound of a ticking clock against a silent backdrop.

There is the ongoing activity of people circulating and a sense that one is private in an otherwise active environment. Surprisingly, this can heighten a sense of quiet, as it is a reminder that others cannot really hear you, for all the outside room distractions. You are tucked away in a quiet room. This contrast may unexpectedly facilitate a feeling of intimacy and encourage the dynamic of disclosure in the course of the therapy hour. Almost a bit like whispering to one's friend in the cinema or theatre, there is a sense that no one else can hear us.

One client, describing how separation from a partner and departure from the family home affected him, was presented with the challenge of adapting to a quieter home life. Reflection on the noise of the children's clinic at the medical centre facilitated the recognition and disclosure of similar sounds missed in the home – the hurley burley of young life carrying on around us. Ultimately, he had disclosed feeling isolated after the break up, and on reflection it seemed that coming into such a busy setting was helpful in breeching that isolation.

Phenomenology of privacy in a public world

It is somehow symbolic of the need for privacy and disclosure in a crowded world that there can be something reassuringly real about it at times. It can be soothing, having this background of life and interaction whilst reflecting on life's experiences and challenges. It is rather like having one's own room in a busy hotel, something people on occasion seek out deliberately. Is it soothing to be connected and disconnected simultaneously, like having the radio on in the background as I type?

One's attitude to the noise of children is often one of tolerance and delight. Some clients' reaction to the surrounding clamour from the children's clinic can on occasion be positive too. I liken it to hearing the rainfall when working at home, or the sound of someone cooking dinner when one is unwell in bed. Occasionally, on a very busy day, other consultants are heard talking, other people are being helped, looked after, babies can be heard in the baby clinic sometimes crying, sometimes playing, children at times run up and down the corridor whilst waiting for appointments.

Therapist and client are immersed in everyday reality. However, there are times when it is extremely quiet too. More so around the COVID-19 lockdown and after, when more practitioners were working from home. Interestingly, it did not seem to have much effect on the therapeutic interaction. Do we perhaps put more emphasis on some of the established benefits to the therapy hour, such as absolute silence, than we need to?

Daily humdrum sounds are also present in the waiting room. The crackling of the coffee machine, and the chatter of secretaries perhaps create a calm and containing environment for clients.

Smells and taste

Sounds, smell and taste are often interlinked. The mechanical drinks machine creates sounds of electrical energy and running liquids, smell and eventually taste. Coffee seems to be therapy friendly, in that it often accompanies clients in to the room often to be followed by expressions like 'Don't mind if I finish my coffee, do you?' I recall a time a client arrived with two coffees fresh from Costa. 'One for me and one for you' they announced. In this unusual moment, we were united by shared experience of taste and smell. I did not finish the coffee as somehow this shared sensual experience induced a feeling of friends chatting over a drink. In the more traditional psychodynamic therapy approach this 'let's be friends and not client and therapist' dynamic would be seen as an incident of transference and/or resistance.

It is however interesting to note the influences of something like a shared beverage. This is perhaps made even more interesting by the curious phenomenon that drinking water, which essentially tastes and smells of nothing, seems to have a neutral impact on the therapy session. Water, and its rather bland taste, does however serve more purpose than a mere refreshment in the session. People who are feeling nervous, perhaps in a first appointment of this kind, may experience symptoms such as a dry mouth. A sip of water can bring immediate relief. Like the aqueous sound of the coffee machine, we hear the sound of water hitting empty cups in the waiting room.

Before proceeding to the role of touch in the therapy setting, it should be pointed out that there is also an interplay between touch and sound. There is the combined experience of sound and touch in the clanking of the computer, as I type out notes in a first appointment undertaking an assessment. This is quite different to the older style of taking notes by hand. The sound is a reminder, and a less subtle one than pen on paper, that we are in a more institutional environment.

Touch

In the morning as I walk in to the practice, I anti-bac my hands as soon as I reach the door. Here there is again an interaction between the senses. The gel smells of antiseptic, alongside the sensation of cooling and cleansing my hands. Once applied, my hands are clean, in harmony with the therapist's neutral, uncontaminated stance, often referred to in the psychodynamic framework as 'the blank slate'. This is perhaps a metaphor for my personal psychological baggage being left at the door of the clinic, alongside the other possible physical contaminators that are wiped away by a squeeze of anti-bac gel onto my hands.

Generally speaking, my working day is free from touch. There is a significant absence of touch in my consulting room. This is in contrast to the doctor's where physical medical examinations are likely to be taking place. Neither is it like physiotherapy or massage where the therapy is mostly physical. Psychological therapy takes place entirely through conversation, sounds and even silence, which can at times scream of various concealed feelings.

Occasionally there may be a touch with the greeting of a handshake, and sometimes this can reveal something about a person. The firm brief handshake can communicate interest and enthusiasm, whilst a very strong one may indicate a dominant or more formal personality. A sense of touch can hint at the client's disposition or feelings about the anticipated psychological counselling experience.

The pandemic regulations forbade touch and in the context of talking therapy where touch is absent from the process, these regulations served to reinforce the absence of physical contact. Talking therapy is the one line of care work where touch is absent, unlike most care work that often involves looking after people's basic needs such as bathing, dressing, lifting, assisting with medication or performing medical examinations or investigations.

Significantly, there is perhaps more self-touching that occurs in my appointments. Some clients twirl their hair and wring their hands; feelings are communicated through visible tactile tensions or acts of self-soothing. Other more tender emotions can be conveyed too by a hand on the heart or the gesture of a prayer, perhaps more likely to be displayed from those of more emotionally demonstrative nationalities and cultural backgrounds.

Sixth sense

Having reflected on the therapeutic manifestations of the five senses, I will consider the presence of what is often referred to as the 'sixth sense'. This is a power of perception frequently thought of as analogous to sense, perhaps an intuitive power.

First impressions are important in the work of therapy and we are encouraged to explore them. Such impressions and instincts often operate through a process known as transference. Transference occurs when someone redirects their feelings about one person onto someone else. During a therapy session, it usually refers to a person transferring their feelings about someone else onto their therapist. Conversely, countertransference is when a psychologist transfers feelings from their personal relationships onto the patient. This concept of countertransference is complex and widely written about in psychoanalytic theory and has also been at the heart of theoretical debates and clinical practice within both psychotherapy and psychology (Boden, 2021).

The concept of transference was first described by psychoanalyst Sigmund Freud in his book *Studies on Hysteria* (Breuer & Freud, 1955). It is mostly an unconscious experience that psychodynamic therapy would wish to make conscious. This sense of intuition may reflect the mind's need to sense and process what may happen next. Client and therapist may therefore make assumptions about each other when they first meet and this reflects the presence of a sixth sense in the therapy sessions. Sometimes, a client's personality traits may be revealed by the distance they keep. Some clients pull their chair right up to the front of the table, and rest their arms on it while talking. This more forthcoming personality likes to get close up, whilst others lean back in a chair, set a few feet back from the desk, sometimes more remote and reflective in character. These are perceptions and interpretations of clients triggered by the therapist's intuition at the time. Here we are understanding and interpreting people through our gut feeling and not through what they are telling us.

Intuition and gut feeling often referred to as the sixth sense reflects an ability to detect pain, empathy and often what is going on for our clients, as they sit in the space with us. Sometimes when someone is frozen and says nothing, we are able to pick up what might otherwise be said in words, without them. In such instances, one could say that we rely on our 'sixth sense' in psychological counselling.

How the medical setting can influence attitude to therapy, and if people will have it

The preceding discussion may give rise to the general question: How much does the therapeutic environment *matter* in the psychological counselling setting?

There was a time where I straddled two different clinical environments that were in direct contrast with each other. One being the medical setting described previously and the other the traditional quiet, comfortable room, complete with armchairs, pretty wallpaper, a beautiful clock and table and a large window opening onto a tree-lined sky. It struck me how unaffected my clients were by these apparently opposite environments, when they might come from one clinic to the other. Surprisingly, the different environments were rarely mentioned and when they were, disappointment was seldom communicated. The odd comment such as 'Oh! This is a different setting, much more clinical' almost seemed irrelevant once the client had spotted their seat, got comfortable and began to talk to me.

It would appear in these different settings the common denominator was me, the counselling psychologist. This highlights the centrality of the therapeutic relationship that can be transferred to more than one setting once the psychological counselling is established and clients feel secure. This is perhaps even more apparent now with the recent development of online therapy sessions since COVID-19. In such instances there is no shared therapy room at all.

It is a common occurrence, particularly in the central London private medical arena, that people come from abroad for medical treatment. Some come from as far as the Middle East. Although the trips are often initially for medical treatment purposes, a desire for all the additional treatments that happen to be on offer can emerge. This can activate a somewhat 'supermarket' approach. Time may be spent sitting in waiting rooms in between appointments observing and absorbing what is going on around them. A list of consultants and their area of expertise is on display that can trigger an interest and enthusiasm for additional alternative appointments not previously considered or even required.

I have had people come to see me who, having noted my stated skills, seemed to think it was a good idea. Interestingly, such an impromptu attendance often makes for a brave and interesting presentation, which can act as an immediate and cathartic release for someone from another culture where such an opportunity is limited, not least due to the social stigma related to attendance. Satisfaction and enthusiasm are often then communicated to family members, who can also decide capriciously to attend an appointment with me too. In such instances, therapy continuation online is often requested. One could term this 'self-referral by situational opportunity'.

Because the way I work is more in line with the way a medical general practitioner works, clients book their appointments whenever they see fit, 'as and when'. Sometimes a number of sessions are agreed to in advance, as is often the case when clients have authorisation from insurance companies for six to twelve sessions and sometimes more.

This approach encourages regularity of attendance. It also encourages people to attend only when in need even if it is only once or twice, to get on top of a particular issue at the time. This approach is at odds with the older traditional psychodynamic approach of seeing clients sometimes two or three times a week on a weekly basis, for an unlimited period of time. Regular attendance however can be arranged for those who book sequential appointments up front.

This approach of 'as and when' booking is sustained and perhaps reinforced by the large reception area where secretaries book appointments. There is a clear and visible separation between myself as the psychologist and the reception booking area. If someone leaves and does not want to rebook, they can leave discreetly without any further discussion of why they won't be booking their next appointment.

It could be argued this has advantages and disadvantages. My relationship with the client can be independent of bookings, appointments and payment process. This creates a level of client autonomy around attendance and possible therapy termination, unlike the more traditional psychodynamic approaches where any issues would be identified, named, encapsulated and explored within the therapeutic relationship.

Working in a medical setting as a psychologist can encourage clients to sometimes perceive the therapist as a medical doctor too. I have found that when working in a doctor's room in a medical centre, clients are more inclined to disclose and present with physical symptoms as well. This is not only restricted to private practice, as this was evident too when I was working in N.H.S. hospitals and G.P. surgery settings. It seems more likely there will be an assumption that I will know exactly what illness they are experiencing and describing, and any taken treatments. Though I have extensive knowledge of the medicines prescribed for psychological disorders, this is not extended to all physical illness. It seems there is a strong association some clients make with the medical doctor behind the desk that at times has to be dismantled and related expectations minimised and managed.

Further clinical benefits of providing psychological counselling in a medical setting

Bullmore (2022) cited that we live in a divisive world where a hard line is drawn between mental and physical health. He claims that the deeply entrenched distinction is disadvantageous to patients on both sides of the divide. He goes on to say that psychological symptoms in patients with physical disease are disabling and undertreated. On the other hand, the physical health problems in people suffering psychiatric disorders contribute to a reduced life expectancy.

One of the great advantages of offering psychological counselling in a medical setting is the presence of the multidisciplinary team. There is an environment of extensive medical and healthcare services on offer. Various consultants such as endocrinologists, dermatologists, cardiologists, ophthalmologists, paediatricians, dieticians, physiotherapists, general practitioners and nurses are in immediate circulation.

There is the benefit of cross referral, and if consent is given, client discussion from various professional health care perspectives. This can help when there may be physical aspects and/or symptoms of illness and/or disease in clients' presentations and difficulties. There are also occasions where the psychologist may feel there is comorbidity and the client is suffering from possible physical symptoms of a condition too.

An example of this is a client of mine who presented with acne-related distress and weight gain, which she described as being uncontrollable. She also disclosed a pronounced disruption to her monthly cycle. The presentation was sounding familiar to the symptoms of polycystic ovary syndrome. Upon mentioning this to her, she had not heard of the condition. As I explained what I knew of it, she became interested and readily identified with the symptoms we read together on the N.H.S. website.

She then decided that she would like to see one of our endocrinologist consultants to investigate further. I was able to refer her to an established colleague and it transpired she was suffering symptoms of the syndrome and went to undergo appropriate treatment. This helped her recover not just psychologically but physically too, which furthermore helped reduce any related emotional distress. Sometimes, medical consultants feel patients' symptoms are being exacerbated by stress or occasionally may be psychosomatic. Again, it is helpful that in such instances they can make a direct referral to me for a psychological assessment and sometimes ongoing therapy.

There have also been occasions where clients have been referred to me by doctors, who subsequently are seen to be suffering from conditions such as depression or anxiety. They may or may not be already under medication. This is similar to the referral process from psychiatrists. Again, we get the interactive and joint reflection when consent is given, and this can be very helpful to therapy outcome. It also helps to receive the initial psychiatric assessment in such cases providing valuable insight into the problem.

The medical setting also provides the setting for systemic therapy where the interventions are targeted towards a group, such as a family, as opposed to the individual. An example of this is a child who has been diagnosed with diabetes. Such a situation will impact the whole family and often therapy is required to help them all adjust and adapt. Working in a medical centre amongst many diabetes specialists and endocrinologists allows shared care and systemic intervention in such cases. Here holistic support can be offered.

Conclusion

One might ask the question, is the medical setting ultimately a healing space for psychological therapy? Success of therapy overall amounts to reduction of emotional distress, symptoms of psychological disorders such as panic attacks, anxiety, stress and depression to name a few. Helping clients resolve their presenting problems, resulting in improved quality of life, feeling happier and making decisions and desired changes, are all indicative of success in therapy. Perhaps the most obvious indicator is completion of therapy, when the client no longer feels the need to attend, as their difficulties and related distress are resolved. However, some clients may reappear, if new difficulties or challenges occur.

The previous examples of therapeutic success are all ones seen in a medical setting. In my own professional experience, having worked both in medical settings and more traditional cosy and comfortable consulting rooms, there has been no difference in levels of reported and witnessed therapeutic client outcomes, as documented previously. One might therefore conclude that therapy in a medical setting is as effective as therapy in the more traditional counselling room. It would therefore seem reasonable to assume that the therapy relationship can be the key factor in therapy success and that this does not necessarily require a cosy and soft environment.

References

Adshead, G., & Holmes, E. (2021). *The devil you know: Encounters in forensic psychiatry*. Faber & Faber.

Andrade, C. C., & Delvin, A. S. (2017). Do the hospital rooms make a difference for patients' stress? A multilevel analysis of the role of perceived control, positive distraction, and social support. *Journal of Environmental Psychology, 53*, 63–72.

Boden, M. D. (2021). *Narrative analysis narrative analysis* [Doctor of psychology (PsychD), University of Surrey]. https://doi.org/10.15126/thesis.900114

Breuer, J., & Freud, S. (1955). *Studies on hysteria (1895)* (Standard ed., Vol. 2). Hogarth Press.

Bullmore, E. (2022). *The big idea. Should we drop the distinction between mental and physical-health*. Retrieved September 12, 2022, from www.theguardian.com/books.

De Angelis, T. (2019). Better relationships with patients lead to better outcomes: A good relationship is essential to helping the client connect with, remain in and get the most from therapy. *American Psychological Association, 50*(10).

Nasar, J., & Devlin, S. A. (2011). Impressions of psychotherapist offices. *Journal of Counselling Psychology, 58*(3), 310–320.

5 Unfurling Ariadne's thread
Psychic connections and the engagement of the 'sixth sense' in the consulting room

Christina Moutsou

Introduction

A patient brings a dream featuring my daughter and my husband, her description of them uncannily accurate. I experience a numb ache in the first assessment session with a patient who later informs me of disease precisely on that site of his body. Memories of past trauma surface for a patient at the time I have begun recognising and processing similar events in my own life. Another patient brings a dramatic story set in a part of the world I am about to visit for my holiday the following week. How does the space of the consulting room hold a conversation that entails unconscious connections and the reeling out of threads that neither the therapist nor the patient can fully grasp? Could it be argued that such threads compose the fabric of the therapeutic journey for both parties?

What is the so-called sixth sense, and if we were to profess that it does exist, how does it relate to the space of the consulting room? Could we, for example, have the same degree of intuition and unconscious connection through online work and in relation to patients that we have not met in person? In reality, and as discussed in other chapters of this book, there are more than five senses that constitute the realm of human experience. Also, and perhaps most importantly, our perception of relationships within space is synesthetic, i.e., it is the result of all our senses combined and more.

The term sixth sense has been formulated within materialist theory to convey what is not easy to define in human connection as opposed to the other five more concrete senses (Walton, 2016). Walton is critical of the sixth sense, which he describes as telepathy, the ability to guess what others think, as opposed to our perception based on what we can see, hear, smell, taste and touch, though he accepts that inner processes such as phantasy, imagination and memory are crucial in our perception of the world (Ibid, 2016). In his view, a theory of the senses provides a contrast to idealism and the mind–body duality, which is based on theorising and abstraction, while the sixth sense goes against the grounding realm of bodily experience (Ibid, 2016).

DOI: 10.4324/9781003346845-7

One of the most pivotal and persistent schisms within the history of psychoanalysis has been between Carl Jung, whose clinical work and writings had as a central focus religion, spiritualism and psychic phenomena as part of such traditions, and Sigmund Freud, who insisted that psychoanalysis was a science and a branch of medicine (Kerr, 2011). Though placing sixth sense phenomena in the consulting room within the area of spiritualism and metaphysics is not my aim in the present chapter or my personal inclination, Carl Jung's concepts of the collective unconscious and of telepathy and prophesy as, for example, applied in social dreaming matrix work (Clare & Zarbafi, 2019) are significant aspects of what I see as psychic phenomena in the therapy consulting room.

In my experience, intuition and even phenomena, which are closer to what has been described as clairvoyance and/or telepathy, are part of our embodied connections in significant relationships and they are not uncommon, though they are certainly under-theorised, overlooked and downplayed within psychoanalytic theory, as a result of the previously mentioned historical split at its roots. Within Freudian psychoanalysis, a link has been made between such psychic phenomena and psychosis and borderline phenomena (Klein, 1946; Rosenfeld, 1987), in the sense that such phenomena are seen as preceding the formation of language (what we can speak about and therefore make conscious). Though I would agree that a predisposition to psychic connections may be an attempt to connect with preverbal experience and a sense of fusion with the Mother's body on a psychic level (Searles, 1979), I would argue that the censoring of such phenomena and their representation within classic psychoanalysis as a form of madness may be linked with our collective sociocultural fear and suspicion of fusional states of mind and the longing of union with the Mother (Mayo & Moutsou, 2016).

Freud, despite his deep suspicion of religion and its links with spiritualism, attempted to conceptualise psychic phenomena in his paper, *The Uncanny* (Freud, 1919). Freud lists a number of supposedly supernatural phenomena, such as ghost viewing, live speaking dolls, doppelgängers, etc., and demonstrates how they are all triggered by infantile anxiety as part of the pre-oedipal and oedipal stages of development and how they can persist in adult life through the lifting of repression and repetition compulsion (Ibid, 1919). Following the Freudian tradition, many debates within contemporary post-Freudian psychoanalysis, especially by therapists and theoreticians who work with the more extreme spectrum of mental disturbance, have included in their discussions of countertransference what we understand as psychic phenomena. This is most frequently seen as unconscious communication from the patient who is in the paranoid–schizoid state of mind (Lindner, 1955).

How can we conceptualise the aforementioned phenomena within the space of the consulting room? I do not think that such psychic communication is necessarily restricted in in-person encounters, but the triadic relationship of therapist, patient and the container of the consulting room such as in the notion of two embodied subjectivities meeting in space, whether virtual or physical, may help us understand how such phenomena unfold. In this sense, the consulting room can be the field for the interplay of mutual perceptions between the therapist and the patient including the possibility of tuning into unknown territories of each other's psyche.

Psychic connections in the consulting room: a case of projective identification or a relational premise?

Though the mystical links of the concept of the sixth sense are still frowned upon within psychoanalysis, especially in the circles that profess that psychoanalysis is of scientific validity, at the core of object relations theory is the concept of *projective identification*. In projective identification, the patient places inside the therapist parts of their experience that are so unprocessed that cannot be tolerated (Rosenfeld, 1987).

> Peter[1] announces at the beginning of the session that he heard his mother is in a comma after an accident. Peter has been estranged from his mother through being able to name in therapy the lasting and damaging abuse he has endured by her. His mother has always lived a reckless life fuelled by addiction. I say it is shocking to hear. He corrects me. He says it is NOT shocking at all to hear, it is the expected outcome of the way she has lived her life! Of course, Peter is right, but he sounds very rational and composed, logical and measured in his reaction. Am I then left to carry the part of the frightened, confused child at the mercy of an abusive mother who will now be left with nobody to take care of him? Is this child in him deeply shocked? My uttering seems to communicate the disavowed feeling that should perhaps have been contained by me for now.

I was vehemently opposed when sitting my training thesis viva by two examiners with Kleinian sensibilities who seemed rather dismayed that the main premise of my dissertation was arguing against the concept of projective identification. My central argument was that we are relational beings in constant fluidity between the inner and the outer as well as the space in between us. What material is it that engages our deep intuition and how, and even more importantly in relation to the subject matter of this book, how does the intersubjective space of therapy harbour such intuitions? The concept of projective identification implies that there is a doer and a done to (Benjamin, 2017) and that in such a claustrophobic and exclusive dyadic relationship, the therapist offers her psyche, almost in a victimised state, in order to contain the unprocessed toxic material of the patient. The consulting room though, literal or virtual, can provide a third space for the interaction of the material between the two parties, and as described in the architectural chapters of this book, it can provide a canvas that invites free association for both.

> In situations of ab-use by a parent, that parent looms large in the child's psychic landscape violently occupying their mental space. In the online sessions with Peter, the camera is switched off on his request. The intimate voice-to-voice contact transports me to his haunted psychic landscape and to my own past experiences of possession by a parent. There is no common space to use for free association other than each other's voice, a familiar dyadic enclose.
>
> My father was the kind of man who would ab-use others' space including my own, as he had a deep need to be carried and contained, to get under people's skin. I remember how shocked I was when he lay unconscious just an hour before his death, as at that moment, he could finally no longer creep in. I knew from my own past therefore how strange and shocking it feels not to be occupied and possessed by the very person we have been preoccupied with for all our lives.

The unthought known

The *unthought known*, a term formulated by Christopher Bollas (2017) as an attempt to integrate Freudian theory with object relations, describes well in my view the unconscious interplay between people and the effects of repression on the psyche. I think this could also provide us with an important alternative understanding of sixth sense phenomena in the consulting room. What is it that we cannot consciously acknowledge about each other and yet have a profound sense of well before it becomes conscious?

> One of my first long-term patients, Celia, a middle-aged woman who was struggling with the emotional distancing of her husband, started lying on the couch after the first year of therapy in order to try and minimise her need to stare at me, something we had both recognised as an anxiety response about what, if anything, I could give her that would be helpful to her. At this stage in the therapy, she was complaining intensely about the state of her relationship and was struggling to communicate her frustrations with her husband. It was after a couple of sessions when she lay down on the couch

that I had an anxious dream where I was telling my patient that it must be hard to tolerate that her husband was messing around.

I took this dream promptly to supervision. My supervisor asked me if I had consciously thought that my patient's husband may be cheating on her and went on to comment further on my patient's material. I interrupted him for clarification, as I could not follow. As English is my second language, I was not aware of this particular meaning of 'messing around', at least not on a conscious level. He confirmed that messing around in English also means cheating! The thought that my patient's husband may be having an affair had not crossed my mind up to that point, but I certainly kept it in mind as a possibility after taking my dream to supervision. A few months later, this is exactly what transpired when Celia's husband disclosed to her that he had a relationship with another woman and that he wanted a divorce!

This dream can be seen as an example of Bollas's notion of the 'unthought known'.

My patient must have been suspecting her husband's affair at the time I had the dream, but she was not emotionally able to confront her gut feeling, which was unconsciously communicated to me. Lying on the couch reduced her anxiety about the sessions, and this unconscious material was communicated through right brain to right brain activity as highlighted by Amid and Bachar (2022). Even after having the dream, it is possible that the unconscious communication would have remained concealed was it not for my supervisor's intervention. This is also an example of how repression operates. Difficult feelings only come to light when we are able to begin facing up to them. In the context of embodied therapy within space though, it may be that one of the two parties of the relationship, the therapist, needs to contain the patient's emotional reality until the latter is able to confront it more directly.

The sixth sense was something I often discussed with my long-term training therapist. She had shared with me that she too had experienced psychic connections with patients, especially in the early years of her practice. I had found this very helpful, as it allowed me to share openly my own multiple experiences of such phenomena with her, especially as, like her, I tended to have more such occurrences in the early years of my practice.

My first long summer break from therapy was particularly challenging, as I was processing loss in my past and fear of loss in my present circumstances. Fear of loss when the trauma has been in the past is often interpreted in analytic work as 'anxiety', as the phantasy of what might be lost in the future invariably refers to what has already taken place. This was also my preferred interpretation, and yet the fear had felt particularly rife that summer. Trauma and death were also present in the collective unconscious of my training organisation, as a senior member had died suddenly in a mountaineering accident leaving his wife and teenage children behind. It would not be far-fetched to suggest that on a group level we were all processing previous experiences of loss and trauma.

In the dream I had that summer somewhere midway during the break from therapy, I had a cat and a dog. The cat was called Alice. They were playing with each other not without expressing some hesitation and suspicion in their interaction. Alice, the cat, suddenly started running away from the dog who had become threatening and in her panic, she ran off the window and fell to her death.

I had sensed that the dream was significant and ominous, confirming my worst fears of imminent loss. It also included imagery connected to the tragic accident of the senior member we were all touched by. I wrote the dream down in my diary and dutifully took it to therapy upon my return. It was during that week back that my worst fear was confirmed, as I was faced with a significant loss in my personal life. In the context of the dramatic events that September, my dream made new sense to me.

When I shared the dream with my therapist, she strikingly asked me about the date I had it. In the following session, she let me know that she had checked her diary and confirmed her memory of a corresponding dream on the day after I had mine. Her disclosure, though not following classic analytic technique, was very helpful in continuing the therapeutic journey after that difficult summer. In her dream, in the incomplete way it has remained in my memory, I had gone to find her to let her know that my cat had just died. I was tearful and devastated, but she could see a whole field full of dead cats and she was trying to tell me about all these other losses in the world.

Reverie

The term reverie has become widely used in psychoanalysis to denote a state of nonverbal parallel communication between the two members of the therapeutic dyad. It is often linked with the therapist's internal free association, if not sometimes apparent absentmindedness, which is an unconscious way of processing the patient's material, and which is reminiscent of the so-called maternal reverie, the mother's ability to tolerate the anxiety that the baby's demands generate in her. Waddell (2002) writes:

> The mother's capacity to hold her baby's anxiety and her own, to go on thinking in the face of puzzling and increasingly intense protest and distress, drawing on and offering her inner resources exemplifies what Bion (1962b) called 'reverie' (p. 36). The mother gradually dispels the baby's distress, seeking to engage with it rather than to explain it. She is able to tolerate not knowing its source.
>
> (Waddell, 2002, p. 33)

The word 'reverie' derives from the French 'rêve', which means dream. Reverie can often create a degree of guilt in the therapist for letting their mind wander. I think that as a term, it highlights the advantage of the embodied therapy in the consulting room for allowing unconscious communication between therapist and patient. As highlighted in other chapters of this book, therapy on screen, especially when face to face with the camera on, is a much more challenging forum for allowing free association for each member of the therapeutic dyad. It has been repeatedly observed that allowing for pause and especially for longer silences is particularly challenging in online, camera-on therapy, and therefore the space for reverie can be shrunk (see Tsogia, Chapter 8 in this volume).

Shortly is an example of reverie, which took place upon my return to in-person therapy with a long-term patient who used the couch before the pandemic and was able to return to it when the rules changed. In this incident, I was able to use the imagery of my reverie directly with my patient, as the length of the therapy journey we had already completed together allowed me to have more trust in the relationship.

> Anna had become particularly worried during the pandemic about the lack of sufficient care that her elderly father was receiving and this was a frequent topic of conversation, sometimes dominating sessions on end. In this particular session, while lying on the couch after a long break of being able to access my room, she was expressing anger and dismay that he was left in his own devices despite clear evidence that his ability to take care of himself was diminished. I sensed that this material was very significant in relation to my patient's history. My mind wandered though and a certain imagery unfolded. I responded acknowledging her anger and sense of helplessness. I reflected back that she felt her father was being put at risk, like a toddler left alone on a high-floor balcony without supervision by bohemian parents who disguised their neglect under the mantra that it would be good for him to play and explore. My response made Anna jump and exclaim 'I can't believe what you just said!' She then recounted her dream of the night before.

In the dream, she was supervising her young son who was playing on a balcony. She noticed there was a large gap between two rails. She told herself that he would know not to go near the gap and then she withdrew her attention and went back in her apartment temporarily forgetting about him. She then heard a loud thud she knew was from her son having fallen off the balcony onto the ground below. She ran downstairs and found him totally deformed, but strangely alive.

I was struck by how identical the imagery in my reverie and in Anna's dream was. Interestingly, in Anna's dream, she was the neglectful parent who pretended it was safe to leave her young son unattended. Her neglect did not cause his death, but permanent damage and deformation nevertheless. Anna's dream made much sense in terms of transgenerational trauma. Her father's mother had died when her father was very young and this had left him, so to speak, with permanent damage. It also made sense in terms of her own repressed aggression and even murderousness. Her father had projected a request for care to her since she was as young as he was when his mother died. This was experienced by Anna as an unbearable psychic burden that she needed to carry throughout her adult life. In her anxiety dream, her murderous wish was expressed through being forgetful, but it was precisely this inattention that filled her with unbearable anxiety and guilt. In other words, Anna found it very difficult to tolerate her anxiety about her father's health and her maternal duties in the way Waddell describes as a state of maternal reverie (Waddell, 2002).

I think that the fact the patient was in the room with me and lying down facilitated our mutual free-flowing access to dream or dreamlike imagery, which transported us closer to a state of reverie as opposed to the catastrophic anxiety depicted in the imagery. However, it was not the first time that I had noticed psychic connections between us. I wonder whether I would have shared the imagery of my reverie, presuming such reverie emerged, if the session was online. I cannot of course be certain about such an alternative scenario, but it seems to me that the physical containment of the room and of Anna lying down on the couch and my bodily proximity besides her created a safe space for the sharing of such delicate material.

And what about prophesy?

Out of all these forms of psychic connections, the one that would probably be met with more resistance as mentioned in the Introduction of this chapter, even within relational psychoanalysis, which has overall moved away from viewing the therapy process as a scientific endeavour, is any phenomenon closer in form to prophesy. The term *synchronicity* was in fact formulated by Jung within the context of his interest in spiritualism and prophesy (Aziz, 1990), but it sits perhaps more comfortably within a professional framework of thinking about how we connect with each other's unconscious material. Synchronicity though, in the way we use it informally as contemporary psychoanalytic jargon, implies a linear sense of time, which is composed of the past (history), the present moment (here and now) and the future (uncertainty). If we were to allow for the notion that time may be more fluid than human societies, especially within the context of western rational thinking, have conceptualised it as, then phenomena that seem to capture a future event (prophesy) could be seen as a form of unconscious communication that can also take place within the therapy relationship. In fact, time is one of the important senses in relation to the consulting room such as in the notion of the time limit of a session, which is most usually the fifty-minute hour and in the sense of the timing of interpretation.

In my twenty-plus years of clinical experience, occurrences that seem to precede meeting a patient, even for the first time, and which accurately predict some of the content of their subsequent communication, are frequent, if not common. For me, they often take the form of a certain mood, a persistent thought, a premonition or sometimes, more concretely a dream that may predispose me to be open to receiving material from that patient. Here is a recent example:

> I wake up for an early start with a clear memory of a dream:
> I am looking for a flat in a stately old building. The building is impressive, but when I go inside, it seems to be dirty and chaotic in its structure. I am then told there is a building nearby that is new and with much better facilities, and which I should visit. This second building has large gardens and even an outdoor swimming pool. I am very surprised to see such block of apartments in London, but wonder whether the swimming pool may prove too cold to swim in, as it is not heated or insulated.
> While getting ready for work, I reflect on the dream and conclude that it may be about a difficult decision I have just made to move from one institution of care to another. My 8 am patient, Iris, my first patient this morning, tells me that she supervised several viewings for prospective buyers of her family house in the last week. Her difficulty and ambivalence about selling her childhood house is familiar material we have been going through for the last year of her therapy. Her family house is in fact an old and historical building in her town. She comes from a wealthy family and both her parents who are now deceased have been implicated with local history. She is telling me how she has to go there early to open the windows and air the space, as some viewers have complained

about the house smelling stale and old. My dream starts acquiring a new meaning in my mind, as though it predisposes me to listen to my patient's familiar material in a new way. I ask if this smell in the house is the smell of death. She says she doesn't think so. She thinks the smell is to do with how old the house is and how many generations of history it has been carrying, including her own birth in that house. We then explore her dilemma in a new way, which is whether she should invest in a project to restore this old historical house or move on to a new project through investing her money to a new flat where she can relocate. We agree that the conflict that she has unconsciously held onto in relation to restoring the old versus investing in the new has been blocking her from being able to move on.

I am thinking of the imagery in my dream, the old stately building whose interior is dirty and chaotic versus the new building with the beautiful gardens and the outdoor cold swimming pool. I realise that in my dream a similar ambivalence is expressed, old, stately, but dark and chaotic versus new, well organised and resourced, but cold. My patient also tells me that she thinks that if she invests in restoring her family house, she will be implicated in old toxicity created by her mother's long-term mental health issues, which she will be unable to resolve, and which are likely to be damaging to her, but if she invests in a new apartment and relocates she will lose some possibly vital connection with her history. It feels like it is the first time that our conversation about her conflict in relation to her family house is leading to some clear thinking and possible resolution.

This is a rather ordinary example of prophetic material, where the imagery in my dream the night before about a difficult dilemma I was facing was very closely connected to the material discussed in the session the morning after. Moreover, the imagery in my dream gave me a clear understanding of my patient's dilemma as well as mine retrospectively. One could argue that my dream was influenced by my unconscious awareness of my forthcoming session with my patient the following morning, but regardless of whether this was an influence or not, the material in my dream was related to a persistent difficult dilemma I was facing that helped me throw light onto my patient's ongoing ambivalence and sense of stagnation. There are more striking examples of prophetic phenomena that have occurred in my life, but the purpose of wanting to acknowledge such occurrences in the consulting room is mainly an attempt to reconceptualise time, as one of the important dimensions of therapy work in the space of the consulting room. It could be argued that time is in fact one of the senses engaged in the therapy relationship within space and that it may be less linear than how it has been envisaged up to now within psychoanalytic theory.

Conclusion: unfurling Ariadne's thread

The so-called sixth sense in the consulting room could be conceptualised like Ariadne's thread, which helps King Theseus navigate the labyrinth and find his way out. The consulting room, to the degree that it acts like a third space that brings together the embodied subjectivities of the two parties of the therapy relationship, can provide the canvas on which such deep unconscious connections unfold. Like the gradual disentanglement of Ariadne's thread that informs Theseus's careful steps out of the labyrinth, such unconscious connections should, in my view, not be dismissed, feared or seen as immature communication from the patient that invade the therapist's psychic space. Like Ariadne, it is the therapist's task to give the patient the ball of thread that will help them navigate their way out of the labyrinth of repetition, compulsion and reenactment. But how can the therapist ever do that without adopting an omnipotent position, as the expert and the professional who knows best what is the right course of action for their patient? The therapist's sixth sense can be conceptualised as precious material that comes to the therapist's awareness, which, when treated with gentleness and respect, can eventually lead both therapist and patient out of the dark labyrinth of their unconscious into light, clarity and a degree of freedom.

Note

1 All names used in clinical vignettes in this chapter are pseudonyms. They all follow the principles of composite case studies (Duffy, 2010).

References

Amid, B., & Bachar, E. (2022). At-one-ment: Beyond transference and countertransference. *Psychoanalytic Perspectives*, *19*(3), 327–347.

Aziz, R. (1990). *CG Jung's psychology of religion and synchronicity*. Suny Press.

Benjamin, J. (2017). *Beyond doer and done to: Recognition theory, intersubjectivity and the third*. Routledge.

Bollas, C. (2017). *The shadow of the object: Psychoanalysis of the unthought known*. Routledge.

Clare, J., & Zarbafi, A. (2019). *Social dreaming in the 21st century: The world we are losing*. Routledge.

Duffy, M. (2010). Writing about clients: Developing composite case material and its rationale. *Counselling and Values*, *54*(2), 135–153.

Freud, S. (1919). The "uncanny". In S. Freud (Ed.), *The standard edition of the complete psychological works of Sigmund Freud, volume XVII (1917–1919): An infantile neurosis and other works* (pp. 217–256). Vintage.

Kerr, J. (2011). *A most dangerous method: The story of Jung, Freud, and Sabina Spielrein*. Vintage.

Klein, M. (1946). Notes on some schizoid mechanisms. *International Journal of Psychoanalysis*, 27, 99–110.

Lindner, R. (1955). *The fifty-minute hour: A collection of true psychoanalytic tales*. Rinehart.

Mayo, R., & Moutsou, C. (Eds.). (2016). *The mother in psychoanalysis and beyond: Matricide and maternal subjectivity*. Routledge.

Rosenfeld, H. (1987). *Impasse and interpretation: Therapeutic and anti-therapeutic factors in the psychoanalytic treatment of psychotic. Borderline, and neurotic patients*. Tavistock.

Searles, H. F. (1979). *Countertransference and related subjects: Selected papers*. International Universities Press.

Waddell, M. (2002). *Inside lives: Psychoanalysis and the growth of the personality*. Routledge.

Walton, S. (2016). *In the realm of the senses: A materialist theory of seeing and feeling*. John Hunt Publishing.

Part 2

Dialogues between architecture and psychoanalysis

6 On the architect's couch
Elective affinities between architecture and psychoanalysis
Korina Filoxenidou and Katerina Kotzia

Introduction

Is the architectural view on the consulting room capable of changing the way psychoanalysts perceive their working place as a means of unutterable communication with the analysand? Towards what direction could the psychoanalysts' interest turn in relation to the shaping of the consulting room, through the prism of an architectural understanding of their choices and decisions, as these are reflected in space?

For the restless architect–researcher, every project in architecture – whether real or hypothetical – brings forth a variety of questions related to the subject of design. In the same way actors, especially those who are not matched to a specific type of role, do not know the character they are going to play in the future, architects, too, are not aware of the subject of design; in fact, the only thing they know beforehand is that the subject will not necessarily resemble any of their past or future projects. Thus, every design project, from a chair to a museum, requires a thorough exploration into the universe of the elements that have already formed any preconceived idea of it.

By the time architects are ready to defend their own decisions on the issues they have been called on to address – through a certain design proposal – they have walked a long way full of multiple possibilities that have been dealt with specific choices. Eventually, regardless of the design approach, their proposal becomes the sum of these choices. For this reason, the questions posed by architects at the preliminary research stage are very crucial because they will lead them not only to get closer to their subject and define the issues at stake, but also to reconsider those issues.

The architectural research perspective is the starting point for a series of thoughts that are elaborated in this chapter and are prompted by the space of the consulting room, as well as by the way stereotypes, taste and time shape this space. Through the juxtaposition of architectural and psychoanalytic practices, we seek to trace a common ground in the thinking, intentions and aims of the two disciplines besides the specific architectural or psychoanalytic methods and approaches. In the case of a hypothetical architectural commissioning on the psychotherapy consulting room, curiosity and interest in the subject of study alongside all the questions that would inevitably arise would be both a prerequisite and a starting point for the design process. At the same time, such a hypothetical commissioning would constitute the perfect opportunity for readers to take a quick glimpse into architectural thinking.

On stereotypes

In the field of architecture, questioning stereotypes is a constant challenge. Through all kinds of representations, the propagation of stereotypes is a fact, and their dominance is self-evident. In this way, the conception of almost every space, from children's rooms to spacecrafts, gets rapidly popularised and crystallised into specific spatial characteristics. The consulting room is no exception to that. From Woody Allen's films (Huerta, 2008) to T.V. series, like *In Treatment*,[1] there is a varied – though limited in range and originality – spectrum of representations of interior spaces that constitute the dominant paradigm of the consulting room: warm-lighted, tidy spaces decorated in an either classic or sophisticated fashion, not too big but neither too small, often including at least one bookcase with lots of books, artwork and a selection of pieces of comfort furniture covered with soft fabrics.

These examples, together with the widespread use of photographs depicting Freud's consulting room (Engelman, 1981) – now transformed into a museum (Austrian Cultural Forum, 2017) that attracts numerous visitors[2] – have vigorously formed a stereotypical image of the psychotherapy consulting room that goes beyond the depiction of just its functional needs, which is for a space with a couch and two seats, one occupied by the analyst and the other by the analysand, who either sits on the chair or lies down on the couch, depending on the stage of the analysis.

A quick search on the internet[3] shows that these stereotypical images have been analysed and interpreted in an arbitrary way, to provide a codified set of guidelines for the creation of a 'proper' consulting room that could be summarised as the following: pastel colours, soft fabrics and art. Similarly, upon browsing Pinterest,[4] one can come across an abundance of cases where the aforementioned recommendations have been put in practice, which in turn perpetuate the stereotypical image of the consulting room, informing the way this space is shaped in the Western world.[5]

Analysts have an arsenal of interpretation tools at their disposal that assist them in approaching the analysand. However, every case is different and unique. One could claim that architecture functions in a similar way. From an architectural point of view, it would be too deterministic to link particular decisions about space with a predicted impact on people's behaviour (Sughito, 2016). Design aims at creating spatial conditions that although they can affect the quality of our lives, they cannot – or should not – predetermine them. Every time a new space is designed an important number of parameters is being taken into consideration, opening up the design process to a variety of possibilities that eventually result in an unprecedented outcome. Just like in the psychoanalytic process between an analyst and the analysand, architects and the space they undertake to shape have something in common: nothing is predetermined.

In this respect, stereotypical recommendations for the consulting room, often presented as a warranty for a sense of comfort, are rather biased and naive. Moreover, they imply that comfort suggests the ideal spatial condition for a fruitful psychoanalytic process. But does the idea of comfort have a universal or indisputable quality, or does it just form another stereotype?

If we are to develop this thought further, it would probably be more interesting to question the notion of *comfort* as a *sine qua non* condition. In this direction, Japan-born artist Arakawa and American poet, writer and philosopher Madeline Gins use their architecture works as a means of protest against the notion of comfort in the space we live and move daily; they, in fact, claim rather provocatively that comfort – as a spatial goal – contributes to the physical hypnosis of the human body.

Arakawa and Gins (2002) introduced a concept they called 'reversible destiny' according to which architecture can put us in a state of emergency through the creation of spaces that challenge the body. Hence, they claimed that design is capable of strengthening the immune system and can help us live longer. In order to test their argument, they designed and implemented various projects in Japan and in the U.S.A.; the Biosclave House[6] (Lifespan Extending Villa) completed in 2008 at East Hampton, New York, is a good example of their work, with a rather peculiar interior that gets visitors in the mood for exploration. The floor is bumpy and there are columns to lean on while moving around the space. Yet, the residences are luminous and spacious, meaning that not every commonly accepted spatial quality has been questioned by the creators. However, one may find more than forty colours in the space and the levels of each room are hard to approach or, perhaps, they can be approached in a rather adventurous way. By converting the disadvantage of a sense of uncertainty – which is felt when wandering around these interiors – into an advantage, the creators' intention was to push through the limits of the prevailing view that considers comfort in space to be an established principle and, therefore, an indisputably desired spatial quality.

In light of this example, and having in mind the fact that each analyst has a unique approach, it might be an interesting idea to question the stereotypes and reconsider the space of the consulting room, allowing more space for experimentation and individual design approaches.[7]

A matter of taste

The word taste[8] is used in English to convey two different meanings. One meaning is related to the physical sense of taste, like sour or salty, sweet or bitter, as well as to other characteristics of the food that we perceive when tasting it in our mouth; the other meaning is related to aesthetic judgement. In Greek, there are two different words for these two notions (γεύση [gefsi] and γούστο [gusto]), yet they originate from the same root, which is the Latin word *gustus*.

French sociologist Pierre Bourdieu (Bourdieu, 1984) talks about the ideological charge of taste (as aesthetic judgement) and establishes how taste is directly linked to the social stratification, while Hegel (Hegel, 1975) already as early as the beginning of the 19th century defines taste as the educated sense of beauty. Therefore, the way we perceive taste is directly linked to culture, both in terms of the intellectual (sociocultural context) and the material (civilisation) world.

Although taste in its aesthetic sense constitutes the most direct criterion for tracing similarities and differences amongst people, it also claims a subjectivity that can bring us to absolute exposure. We express our taste by talking about our preferences, from the performance of the second part of 'Andante ma moderato' of Brahms' Sextet No. 1 to the side we sleep on. Similarly, even in the absence of speech, our taste is manifested through our choices, like the car we drive or the clothes we choose to wear. Hence, our taste is indicative of our identity, and, in this regard, manifesting it requires taking a risk that can enable both differentiation and integration.

In addition to the clothes and other accessories that we choose for our personal presentation, the aesthetics of our space is also an unutterable expression of our taste. Whether it is the interior of our home or that of our working place, 'our' space is a tangible display of the choices we make. Contrary to the clothes we wear or the car we drive that cannot be concealed, we expose our private space selectively.

In light of this and given that in the traditional analyst–analysand relationship, the analyst is not supposed to reveal information about their personal life, one would expect that a consulting room would be a space as *neutral* as possible. Since there is no such concept as *neutral* space – as 'a signifier without signified has no meaning', according to Saussure (Bouissac, 1998), one would expect that the consulting room would be a space as free as possible from the personal choices of the analyst. In other words, one would anticipate an attempt to design the interior space of the consulting room in a 'white noise' way (Summer, 2022) that seeks to erase the traces of the analyst's identity.

Interestingly, however, this does not seem to be the case. Mark Gerald, a psychoanalyst and photographer, took photographs of several consulting rooms all over the world for the purposes of the publication 'In the Shadow of Freud's Couch', which was one of the main inspirations for this chapter. As we observe the elements that form each one of the interior spaces in these photographs (Gerald, 2020) it is difficult not to notice the bold and sometimes even 'loud' decisions made by each one of the analysts featured in the book, regarding the furniture arrangement, colours and decoration of their consulting room. Most of the consulting rooms presented are far from neutral. On the contrary, they seem to have a strong character, which reveals a lot of information regarding the taste of their proprietors. On the other hand, it is quite uncommon for the analysand to reveal similar details about their space.[9]

In traditional psychoanalysis, we tend to view the relationship between the analyst and the analysand as hierarchical and unequal, as it is the analyst's role to set out the frame and boundaries of the relationship, but also it is the analysand who is emotionally exposed, and therefore vulnerable. The analysand reveals themselves while the analyst remains in the shadow. However, with regards to taste and the way it is stated through the analyst's choices that inform the shaping of the consulting room, there is an implicit reversal in the traditional roles, i.e., the analyst is more exposed than the analysand.

While the analysand remains relatively protected in revealing only parts of their aesthetic taste through their presentation, the analyst exposes – to the value judgement of the analysand – their view about the intimate space of the consulting room, that is to say their taste, which consequently reveals an important part of their identity. In this way, the consulting room becomes a niche through which the analysand is able to penetrate into the analyst's idiosyncrasy.

Of course, not all analysts have a private consulting room. Many have to share institutional or medical rooms where they don't have the possibility of arranging and decorating the space according to their views or personal taste. However, when presented with the opportunity for creating their own consulting room, most analysts tend to create a very personal space according to the tradition that was set out by Freud himself (Gerald, 2020). By observing Gerald's photos, one could argue that analysts often tend to incorporate decorative elements in their consulting room that they are personally attached to, thus creating their working place in the way they would do with a totally *personal* space.[10] Perhaps, it would not be so inaccurate to suggest that since analysts cannot reveal details of their personal lives, they tend to unconsciously 'introduce' themselves to the analysands through the space of the consulting room. This builds an unspoken relationship with each one of their analysands even from the beginning of the analytic process.

In architecture, designing a building for a certain client also involves forging a relationship of trust between the architect and the client, since it is rather impossible for a project to progress unless the project recipient's imaginary vision is revealed. This becomes more obvious when designing a private residence, where architects acquire an intimate knowledge of the owner's personal needs and desires – without having to reveal any of their own – which they consequently interpret according to their own design approach. Up to this point of the process, it appears inevitable to fall into the temptation of comparing the architect–client relationship with that of the analyst–analysand.

In architecture, however, the outcome of the interpretation is reflected in the designed space that eventually becomes an alloy of the two parties of the relationship. It is that alloy – formed as a result of this unique dialectical relationship – that in turn reshapes the two parties respectively. At the end of this process, one could find themselves to be dissatisfied with the outcome, as it might not respond to their desires (either those of the architect, or those of the client – or even those of both parties). Since in the design process all possibilities are left open, it will eventually reach a point where the designed space becomes a self-reliant entity. This entity may *outplace* the owners themselves.

An example of this case, demonstrated in a humorous way, can be found in *This Was Not My Dream*, a short film by architect and director Marcio Kogan, whose architecture studio is known for the design of private residential projects. The film features Redux House, a project completed by Kogan in the countryside of São Paulo. It features a couple and the process of their breakup, prompted by the construction of their new house. The husband, in the role of the narrator, describes how the creation of this residence and its style and aesthetics excluded him from the whole process and alienated him from his wife, Susana. During the film, we watch Susana, as she wanders around the interior and exterior spaces of the house in a way that clearly suggests the development of an intimate relationship between her and the newly designed house; a relationship that is deeply satisfying to her.

Human characteristics and qualities of the space are indirectly attributed to the house, thus making it an object of desire for the wife and an object of rivalry for the husband–narrator. In fact, the narration could easily form part of a psychoanalytic session where this rivalry is discussed, and which concludes with the narrator fantasising that his wife Susana will eventually come back into his arms:[11]

> This situation will not last very long. She'll realise that she has been foolish building that sort of house, the absurdity of her passion and love of this house. She will abandon the metallic door frames and come back into my arms. She will not resist; I am certain of this.

Shortly, she will take her eyes off the flat flagstones and Susana will be mine again.

Hosting and time

Architects design spaces that host events and actions. Prominent architect and thinker Bernard Tschumi in *Architecture Concepts: Red is Not a Color*, claims that space is transformed by events and that buildings acquire meaning as soon as something happens in them (Tschumi, 2012). In most cases, these events are defined by the type and function of a building. However – although the design process in architecture follows the articulation of a programmatic expression of the space, which defines its use and its functional diagram – it is not always possible to predict what may happen inside a building or a public space. Moreover, there is a common view that architecture should not seek to determine everything from the beginning, but rather to become a platform where actions can be performed, where interactions with the space are encouraged and where relations among people can develop effortlessly: a platform that allows inclusion, supports diversity and promotes coexistence. This concept was clearly manifested in the latest Biennale of Architecture in Venice, curated by Hashim Sarkis. In his curatorial statement, Sarkis notes that we need a new spatial contract and calls on architects to imagine spaces in which we can generously live *together* (Sarkis, 2021).[12] Thus, it might be fair to say that the architect is a host – or better yet – an *enabler*, who designs the setting that will allow for different possibilities and events to develop.

Respectively, in analogy to the architect, it could be argued that the analyst takes the role of the host as the sessions with the analysand usually take place either in their own consulting room or, as mentioned before, in a shared or institutional consulting room, where the analyst is still the host when conducting sessions. The analyst not only receives and sees the analysand in the consulting room, but also undertakes the task of arranging the recurring sessions[13] and creating the appropriate setting for them in an effort to ensure that both the spatial and the emotional experience will be agreeable to their analysands.

Thus, the consulting room is definitely a place of hosting, both in a literal and in a metaphorical sense. It is a space where the analysands/visitors go to share their intimate thoughts and to explore their inner feelings in a *welcoming* environment. From an architectural perspective, we would argue that finding a balance between clarity and complexity is important in order to create a more agreeable space. A clear space plan with eminent structure and function is fundamental in order to avoid confusion. However, a certain degree of visual stimuli that may be perceived on a later internalisation of the space could contribute to making it more interesting and intriguing.

Probably, this is the reason why most of the spaces that require a profound connection with their users are filled with visual stimuli. Throughout the history of architecture, the ornamented spaces par excellence have been churches, temples and other similar structures of spiritual expression.

The lengthy amount of time spent in those places while keeping still and quiet is compensated by the use of ornamentation that allows for visual stimulation and is capable of evoking memories and contemplation. Just like in the aforementioned example of the churches, the consulting room is also a space where the amount of visual information is directly related to time. The time that each analysand may need in order to perceive, absorb and internalise this information.

As the space needs to be in flow with the analysands' inner world and in search of the ideal balance, it is important to take under consideration that an overloaded space can be overwhelming, if we do not have enough time to spend in it and digest the visual stimuli. On the other hand, an empty space can result in an uninteresting, even frustrating experience, if we must spend time in it without the opportunity of an indulging visual tour (Filippidis, 2006).

Although ornamentation was abandoned in modern architecture and thought of as brutal by some authors, such as in Adolf Loos's 'Ornament and Crime' (Loos, 1998), postmodernism and, recently, meta-modernism (Danilova & Bakshutova, 2021) has reintroduced the use of decorative elements in design, associating them to memory and people's need to connect with the past.

The consulting room rather than a room of action is a room of stillness and reflection. It is the recipient of narratives originating from an-Other, where the action took place somewhere else in some other time. In that sense, the space of psychoanalysis could be paralleled to that of an ancient Greek theatre, where the action is seldom brought on stage (Sommerstein, 2010). On the contrary, it is transmitted to the audience through an elaborate mechanism that involves messengers, narration and divine interventions.

In the psychoanalytic framework, physical actions that take place inside the consulting room are limited to a rather unintentional browsing of its contents, such as the ornaments and other decorative elements found in that space. Thus, the materials, colours, decorative elements, art and other objects found in the space play a very important role. This becomes very evident in the numerous pictures of consulting rooms taken by Mark Gerald for his book *In the Shadow of Freud's Couch*, mentioned earlier in this chapter (Gerald, 2020). Many of the psychoanalysts interviewed for this publication share details about the decorative elements found in their space and their potential function as part of the psychoanalytic process. In some cases, certain elements that comprise the space proved to be efficient conversation starters (Gerald, 2020).

In an online discussion with a group of psychotherapists from the Philadelphia Association on the role of the decorative elements and objects they choose for their consulting room, one of them presented a Klein bottle.[14] According to this trainee psychoanalytic therapist, the mathematical genius of this object proved to be an effective conversation starter in some of his sessions.

If the consulting room is a sensitive and evocative space where action, as stated previously, is limited to the wandering gaze, then the following question arises: could we map this action[15] and/or discover what it involves, so as to gain a deeper understanding of the user's experience of the consulting room? If so, would it be possible to conceptualise the analysand's experience of the consulting room and benefit from the insights we gain in order to design more efficient and welcoming experimental spaces that are open to new possibilities? Could the sensory stimulation triggered by the room's appearance, internal characteristics (i.e., size, orientation, etc.) and other features (i.e., materials, colours, decorative elements, etc.) be influenced by the sense of time?

Due to our relative perception of time (Robin, 2019) its importance cannot be easily explained or articulated. Eye tracking links visual stimulation with time, thus it could be a useful tool for numerous relevant research projects including that of tracking the analysand's gaze through the interiors of the consulting room. However, the sense of the passage of time is a crucial factor for understanding spatial experience. The act of hosting, which as mentioned before is common to both architectural and psychoanalytic practices, warrants that this parameter should always be taken into consideration.

A belief in change

Although it is a common belief that architects design buildings from scratch, many projects that they deal with concern a preexisting building. It is quite common for architects to undertake the restoration and/or adaptive reuse of existing buildings and complexes, the renovation of old apartments and commercial spaces, the redesign of great urban spaces and so forth. Even in the case of creating a new building, there is always a pre-existing surrounding – a context. Understanding and interpreting this context plays a significant role in the research and design process.

Judging from a global tendency towards preservation (Koolhaas & Otero-Pailos, 2014), as manifested in a great number of published architectural projects regarding the adaptive reuse of old buildings all over the world, it might be fair to assume that architects *must* believe in change and improvement. Otherwise, it would be pointless to dedicate so much thinking and so many working hours on redesigning buildings and residential areas that require amelioration. There is a parallel here with psychoanalysis where change, in the way we perceive the word, is at the core of the discipline. Just like the architect, the analyst too believes in change and embraces it. By respecting and trusting their *material*, analysts try to trace the ability of the analysand for change and to help them discover their potential. In both practices, the notion of change and improvement seems to play a significant role.

Restoration and reuse of buildings is not a new tendency. Throughout the history of architecture, historical buildings were adapted in order to acquire new use and meaning (Richards, 2017). In addition, there has always been a special concern for the preservation of historical monuments and other places of cultural importance. There are specific guidelines[16] as well as several institutions[17] entrusted with the duty to record and archive those cases and – most importantly – to advocate for the adoption of the most suitable and respectful techniques to assure their *healthy restoration*. Preserving historical buildings, monuments and places of cultural value is essential for the preservation of historical continuity. It is in this way that our contemporary society is paying tribute to its roots, and that also explains the sensitivity with which we approach such cases of restoration. This concept might suggest another parallel between architecture and psychoanalysis where the acknowledgement of one's *roots* is also very important for the analytic approach.

Of course, there is a lot of criticism regarding our need for maintenance (Vidler, The New York Times, 2001). In several cases, maintenance and restoration have become habitual and almost obsessive. They are sometimes applied not in order to preserve history and produce an interesting new building in line with its roots and history but rather for the sake of maintenance itself that sometimes leads to the creation of hybrid enigmatic buildings. For example, preserving the (or part of the) façade of an old building – a practice called facadism – without taking into consideration its initial purpose, might give us a purely decorative result that disregards the essence of the building under preservation, thus undermining the whole purpose of historical continuity. On the other hand, great examples of preservation and reuse can be found in recent times. Numerous buildings designed by celebrated architects from all over the world have managed to renegotiate our relation to history by producing examples that express different views in accordance or in contrast with the past (Wong, 2016).

Such examples, even though they are open to criticism, constitute case studies that help broaden the discussion around the role of architecture in the preservation of cultural heritage. They also enrich the relevant architectural discourse with new arguments on burning questions, like submission to history or the revival of the past and all the stages of compromise or affiliation to certain ideologies that lie in between.

However, though the cases of preservation related to buildings of historical value and our position towards them are important, noteworthy examples that strengthen the arguments regarding architects' belief in change and amelioration also come from more trivial backgrounds. In contemporary architecture, the tendency for preservation is becoming all the more inclusive. Actually, a lot of architectural examples of adaptive reuse projects are not to be found in buildings of historical value. On the contrary, they concern trivial examples of existing architecture, where the decision to reuse overpowered the decision to demolish. It is almost like a celebration of the banal, where an unimportant building acquires added value, mainly through new architectural design approaches.

One would think that the idea of making use of the existing building stock simply emerges out of necessity. Due to a number of sociopolitical factors, such as the constant shifts in geopolitical conditions, the unpredictable migration of populations, the urban sprawl, the surrender of urban inner-city areas to capitalism, the abandonment of old trades and occupations and the constant growth in the number of people living in large metropolises, there is an ever-growing building stock that claims attention and retouch.

However, a closer look at several prominent examples of contemporary architecture can argue that there are more reasons for preferring to use what is already there to building a new structure from scratch. In fact, the 2021 Pritzker Architecture Prize, one of the most well-known and highly acclaimed architectural prizes,[18] was awarded to Anne Lacaton and Jean-Phillipe Vassal who run together an architecture studio based in Paris. Above all, the studio's works demonstrate a great concern and sensitivity to social issues. The following quote, taken from a short biographical note from the Pritzker Prize website, explains their view on architecture: 'They vowed to never demolish what could be redeemed and instead, make sustainable what already exists, thereby extending through addition, respecting the luxury of simplicity, and proposing new possibilities' (The Pritzker Architecture Prize: Laureates, 2022).

Jean-Phillipe Vassal stated in an interview: 'Working with existing buildings makes economic as well as environmental sense. . . . If we talk about keeping buildings instead of demolishing them, it's the first step towards sustainability; to make sustainable what already exists' (Block, 2021).

Apart from an obvious appeal to reason, like the economic and ecological benefits of maintaining something that already exists (Harper, 2021), we can also observe something more subtle in the words of this expert. It looks like there is a rather humble approach detached from any narcissistic tendency, and a very different stance from what was obvious in the majority of the works that have been created by architects or, better yet, *starchitects* in the last decades. More interestingly, though, Lacaton Vassal's work does not seek to be didactic. On the contrary, it evokes joy and pleasure. It is the pleasure that can only be derived from making good use of and improving what has always been around. 'Just try to repair and just try to add what is missing. You will give much more pleasure than by rebuilding after demolition' (Block, 2021).

Architects believe in change and this belief is gradually becoming more visible and respected in current architecture. This belief becomes a common ground shared with all those who take pleasure in fixing something old or worn out. In order to change something, one must establish a relation to it. A form of dialogue that will assure that there is an understanding of what needs to be changed. This is an interesting parallel between architecture and psychoanalysis, since the relational paradigm in psychoanalysis is based on constructive dialogue and listening/engaging, rather than the position of the expert who knows better.

Luckily enough, there are more and more examples in contemporary architecture that demonstrate sensitivity and a lack of arrogance. The fact that this work is acknowledged by influential institutions shows that a shift in our values is in the making. Studio Assemble, a collective of architects undertaking social projects, engages with the ideas of reuse. A large part of their work deals with interventions in existing parts of the city, giving new use to abandoned buildings and improving seemingly difficult urban areas through inventive and affordable ideas. In 2015, Studio Assemble won the Turner Prize (https://www.tate.org.uk/art/turner-prize), a prestigious award given annually to a British artist. That was the first time such an award for the arts was given to a group of architects, a fact that probably reflects the current social focus on and concern about sociopolitical issues.

The consulting room is the organic space where the analysand is expected to experience changes in their perspective. At the beginning of this project, during a brainstorming session together with two of the contributing psychoanalysts in this book, Anastasios Gaitanidis and Christina Moutsou, we talked about the decorative items they placed in their consulting rooms, in an attempt to define the reasons behind their choices. At some point, one of the participants, Anastasios, mentioned that he had two pictures hanging on the wall of his consulting room, showing two different phases of the house, where his consulting room was located – before and after. At the time he decided to hang them on the wall, he was not conscious about why he had made this choice, but after a while and judging from the reaction of some of his analysands, he was pleased to discover the 'concealed' message about the importance of the history of a site and the possibility for change and improvement that these pictures subtly expressed.

Epilogue

We believe that all the previous observations and parallels that reflect on our view of the consulting room through the vehicle of architectural thinking could generate a reconsidering of this important space, at least by the psychoanalysts themselves, thus shifting their interest to new points of attention. We have attempted to correlate the processes followed in both disciplines (architecture and psychoanalysis) as a way of understanding the important components of psychoanalytic practice, to the extent that this could become a useful tool of communication between the architect and the psychoanalyst for the sake of redesigning and reconceptualising the consulting room. As we attempt to comprehend the Other, we move towards decoding the mechanisms that define the way we respond – as architects – to the Other's needs and to everything else that the Other anticipates from us. Perhaps, this might be yet another common point that both architecture and psychoanalysis share, and which is probably the most difficult to accomplish.

Notes

1. *In Treatment* is an American drama television series for H.B.O. that went live in January 2008. The series is about a psychotherapist, Paul, and his sessions with his patients as well as with his supervisor.
2. The Freud Museum in Vienna: www.freud-museum.at/en/. The Freud Museum in London, which was also the final home of Sigmund Freud: www.freud.org.uk/. A conversation with the directors of these two museums can be found here: www.acflondon.org/events/two-sides-one-coin-freud-museums-london-and-vienna/
3. There are many websites, such as *Zencare* (https://blog.zencare.co/therapist-office-decor-ideas-2021/), as well as companies, such as *Therapy Brands,* which specialise in health care technologies and publish articles offering design and styling tips for the psychoanalyst's office.
4. Numerous posts can be found on Pinterest under tags like 'The Therapist's Office', 'Psychotherapy Office Ideas', 'Therapist Office Decor', etc.
5. In the chapter in this book titled *Hearing Other Voices*, Anastasios Gaitanidis refers to the consulting room as an *air-tight therapeutic container* – shaped by the dominant discourse – that he needed to *bracket off,* in order to connect with his analysand.
6. Information about this project can be found in this link: www.reversibledestiny.org/bioscleave-house-lifespan-extending-villa/ypo
7. In Korina Filoxenidou and Natalia Varfi's chapter 'Dialogues between architecture and psychotherapy: revisiting four psychotherapy rooms', an individual design approach is attempted in four case studies of consulting rooms.
8. 'Taste' *Merriam-Webster.com*, 2022. www.merriam-webster.com (8 November 2022).
9. The universality of this fact became even more evident during the time of the recent pandemic, as the use of online sessions reversed this dynamic, and therapists started getting a glimpse into parts of their analysands' personal space. Dora Tsogia's chapter 'The screen therapy room: real

flowers in a digital vase' includes several examples of the revealing of the analysands' personal space in online therapy and its implications.
10 This is also evident in a postgraduate research project on the psychotherapy consulting room conducted by Natalia Varfi whose chapter 'Dialogues between architecture and psychotherapy: revisiting four psychotherapy rooms', co-authored with Korina Filoxenidou, is also part of this publication. Natalia, prior to the diploma project that is featured in the aforementioned chapter, contacted a small scale research project for which she gathered more than sixty questionnaires from a corresponding number of analysts and students of psychoanalysis. Most of the responders made specific mention of the importance of the inclusion of personal items and objects in their ideal consulting room.
11 The video can be accessed in the following link: https://vimeo.com/96252361
12 Spaces like the ones that Anastasios Gaitanidis in the chapter 'Hearing other voices' seeks for a consulting room addressed the minority voices of a *vanished* working class.
13 The time spent in the consulting room is limited to approximately fifty minutes. Appointments are usually arranged on the same day of the week and, more often than not, at the exact same time. Although these recurring meetings seem to provide the psychoanalytic process with a sense of structure, the short length of time of each visit/session does not encourage familiarisation with the space. However, due to the recurring character of these visits and the long-term nature of the psychoanalytic journey, it is possible that familiarisation will develop through repetition and – since therapy requires a substantial amount of time commitment in the analysand's life (Kaplan, 2016) – repetition can be a key factor in relating with the space.
14 The Klein bottle (Freiberger, 2015) is a concept introduced by mathematician Felix Klein. Being a non-orientable surface, the Klein bottle has neither an inside nor an outside, it is just one-sided. For example, an ant could walk around on it forever, without ever encountering a boundary or falling over an edge.
15 There is a relevant study that seeks to reveal how we view architecture and particularly the architectural facades through eye tracking (Sussman & Ward, 2017).
16 A key text with guidelines for the conservation and restoration of monuments and sites is *The Venice Charter*. It was drawn up by a group of conservation professionals during the Second Congress of Architects and Specialists of Historic Monuments in Venice, organised by the International Council of Monuments and Sites (I.C.O.M.O.S.), May 25th – 31st 1964.
17 Some of the organisations dedicated to the preservation of historical monuments are:

- I.C.O.M.O.S., a nongovernmental international organisation dedicated to the conservation of the world's monuments and sites.
- U.N.E.S.C.O., an international organisation granting legal protection to the World Heritage Sites, which are landmark buildings and/or areas all over the world that have been designated for protection for their cultural, historical, scientific or other form of significance.
- D.O.C.O.M.O.M.O. International, a nonprofit organisation whose acronym stands for International Committee for Documentation and Conservation of Buildings, Sites and Neighborhoods of the Modern Movement.

18 The Pritzker Architecture Prize is awarded each year to a living architect 'whose built work demonstrates a combination of those qualities of talent, vision and commitment, which has produced consistent and significant contributions to humanity and the built environment through the art of architecture' (www.pritzkerprize.com/about).

References

Arakawa, S., & Gins, M. (2002). *Architectural body: Modern and contemporary poetics*. University Alabama Press.

Assemble Studio: About. (χ.χ.). Ανάκτηση October 13, 2022, από Assemble Studio: https://assemblestudio.co.uk/about

Austrian Cultural Forum. (2017, June Thursday). *Austrian cultural forum*. Ανάκτηση October 21, 2022, από www.acflondon.org/events/two-sides-one- coin-freud-museums-london-and-vienna/

Bachelard, G. (1958). *The poetics of space*. Boston Press.

Block, I. (2021, March 19). *Dezeen: Magazine*. Ανάκτηση October 13, 2022, από Dezeen: www.dezeen.com/2021/03/19/jean-philippe-vassal-pritzker-prize-interview/

Bouissac, P. (1998). *Encyclopedia of semiotics*. Oxford University Press.

Bourdieu, P. (1984). *Distinction: A social critique of the judgement of taste*. Harvard University Press.

Danilova, E., & Bakshutova, D. (2021). Metamodernism: The phenomenon of memory as part of an architectural concept. In *3rd international conference on architecture: Heritage, traditions and innovations* (σσ. 140–146). Atlantis Press.

Engelman, E. (1981). *Berggasse 19: Sigmund Freud's home and offices, Vienna, 1938: The photographs of Edmund Engelman*. University of Chicago Press.

Filippidis, D. (2006). *Anthology of texts of Greek architecture 1925–2002*. Melissa.

Freiberger, M. (2015, January 6). Ανάκτηση November 10, 2022, από Plus. Bringing Mathematics to Life: https://plus.maths.org/content/introducing-klein-bottle

Gerald, M. (2020). *In the shadow of Freud's couch: Portraits of psychoanalysts and their offices*. Routledge.

Harper, P. (2021, March 17). *Dezeen: Magazine*. Ανάκτηση October 13, 2022, από Dezeen: www.dezeen.com/2021/03/17/lacaton-vassals-pritzker-architecture-prize-opinion/

Hegel, G. W. (1975). *Aesthetics: Lectures on fine art* (T. M. Knox, Trans.). Clarendon Press.

Huerta, M. F. (2008). The Cinema as therapy: Psychoanalysis in the work of Woody Allen. *Journal of Medicine and Movies*, 4, 17–26.

Kaplan, M. (2016, August 31). *New York Post: Lifestyle*. Ανάκτηση November 2, 2022, από New York Post: https://nypost.com/2016/08/31/how-long-should-you- really-stay-with-your-therapist/

Koolhaas, R., & Otero-Pailos, J. (2014). *Preservation is overtaking us*. Columbia Books on Architecture and the City.

Loos, A. (1998). *Ornament and crime*. Ariadne Press.

The pritzker architecture prize: Laureates. (2022). Retrieved October 13, 2022, από The Pritzer Architecture Prize: www.pritzkerprize.com/laureates/anne-lacaton- and-jean-philippe-vassal

Richards, C. (2017, January 2). Ανάκτηση November 1, 2022, από The Conversation: https://theconversation.com/reinventing-heritage-buildings-isnt-new-at-all-the- ancients-did-it-too-70053

Robin, L. (2019, Summer). *Stanford encyclopedia of philosophy archive*. https://plato.stanford.edu/archives/sum2019/entries/time-experience/

Sarkis, H. (2021). *How will we live together? Theme of the Biennale architettura 2021*. Retrieved December 10, 2021, από www.labiennale.org/en/architecture/2021/statement-hashim-sarkis#:~:text=The%20Biennale%20Architettura%202021%20is,to%20take%20on%20these%20challenges

Sommerstein, A. H. (2010). Violence in Greek drama. Στο A. H. Sommerstein (Ed.), *The tangled ways of Zeus: And other studies in and around Greek tragedy* (σσ. 30–46). Oxford University Press.

Sughito, E. (2016, August 9). *Medium*. Retrieved October 15, 2002, from Medium: https://medium.com/@social_archi/architectural-determinism- 583fcbb86501#:~:text=Architectural%20determinism%20(sometimes%20called%20e nvironmental,people%20behave%20in%20a%20space

Summer, J. (2022, October 7). Retrieved October 29, 2022, από Sleep Foundation: www.sleepfoundation.org/noise-and-sleep/white-noise

Sussman, A., & Ward, J. M. (2017, November 27). *Common edge: Essays*. Retrieved November 1, 2022, από Common Edge: https://commonedge.org/game-changing- eye-tracking-studies-reveal-how-we-actually-see-architecture/

Tschumi, B. (2012). *Architecture concepts: Red is not a color*. Rizzoli.

Vidler, A. (2001, August 12). Retrieved July 16, 2022, from The New York Times: www.nytimes.com/2001/08/12/weekinreview/ideas-trends-modern-preservation-it-s-still-all-about-form-and-function.html

Wong, L. (2016). *Adaptive reuse: Extending the lives of buildings*. Birkhäuser.

7 Dialogues between architecture and psychotherapy
Revisiting four consulting rooms

Korina Filoxenidou and Natalia Varfi

Introduction

The following work was initiated for the purposes of a diploma project in the department of architecture of the University of Ioannina. The project began in early 2020 and was presented in the department in June 2022. During this time, we all experienced a global pandemic, which marked the beginning of a shift in the notion of the workspace. In order to guard public safety most institutions and also both public and private companies promoted remote labor, which resulted in turning our homes into work environments. Therapy sessions haven't remained unaffected by this change and most of them moved to the intangible online universe. This major shift naturally played a role in the way the project was conducted and enriched the research process with new questions regarding online therapy sessions.[1] Moreover, it provided the researcher with opportunities for opening up the dialogue to an array of professionals that would be more difficult to reach in the pre-COVID era. The four case studies that will be examined in this chapter involve therapists that live and work in Greece and in the U.K.

A research project regarding the space of the psychotherapy consulting room was undertaken prior to this diploma project. The project was conducted through gathering data from anonymous questionnaires handed to approximately sixty qualified therapists and students of psychotherapy. It also incorporated interviews and historical references to Freud's consulting room.[2] One of the main textbooks referred to was Mark Gerald's book *In the Shadow of Freud's Couch: Portraits of Psychoanalysts and their Offices*.

The aim of the initial research project was to explore in what way the structuring of the psychotherapy consulting room space and the narratives behind its interior design choices can be related to the process of psychotherapy. The hypothesis was that the space itself could potentially play an important role in the process affecting both the therapist and the patient. The research thesis highlighted the importance of the

DOI: 10.4324/9781003346845-10

space of the consulting room and the fact that there is a very limited number of references regarding the interiors of therapists' offices. The most intriguing question that came up was 'how should we approach this space in a hypothetical commission?' This question marked the beginning of the diploma project explored in this chapter.

Four psychotherapy consulting rooms became the case studies of the project. Each of them belonged to a qualified practising therapist who consented to participate in this speculative journey. The therapeutic approach of each one of the therapists was the starting point of the discussion. From the beginning of this project, there was a dilemma regarding the space that would be chosen for the implementation of the design ideas that would emerge. Should it be the original space that the therapist is using or an ideal space with locational flexibility and limited to no dimensional restrictions? After a few intense brainstorming sessions, the idea of using the existing consulting rooms of four of the therapists who participated in the research seemed more alluring, as any spatial limitations that would eventually emerge could be taken as an opportunity for a more challenging design approach. The project was built through an open dialogue between the architect and each one of the participant therapists. This dialectic process is standard in a typical architectural project. The feedback that was given in stages as the architectural proposal evolved, was documented and presented along with the final plans, sketches, diagrams, models and three-dimensional representations. The concept behind the documenting of this dialogue was to highlight how fruitful and substantial the exchange of ideas was and how every new sketch became the vehicle that took the dialogue to a deeper level. Following is a presentation of the four cases of psychotherapy consulting rooms.

Transition

Case study 1: Eleni/Thessaloniki, Greece[3]

First meeting

Eleni is practising body psychotherapy. Her practice is housed in a room inside her spacious apartment. The apartment is located on a quiet street, minutes away from the centre of Thessaloniki. Her consulting room is quite small. However, it is relatively high ceilinged and filled with natural light as there is a glass door leading to a small balcony. The room is decorated in bold colors. The walls are painted mint green and the sheer curtains are bright orange. There is a mattress with a light blue throw on it and some wooden furniture. There is also a set of armchairs for sessions that do not require physical involvement.

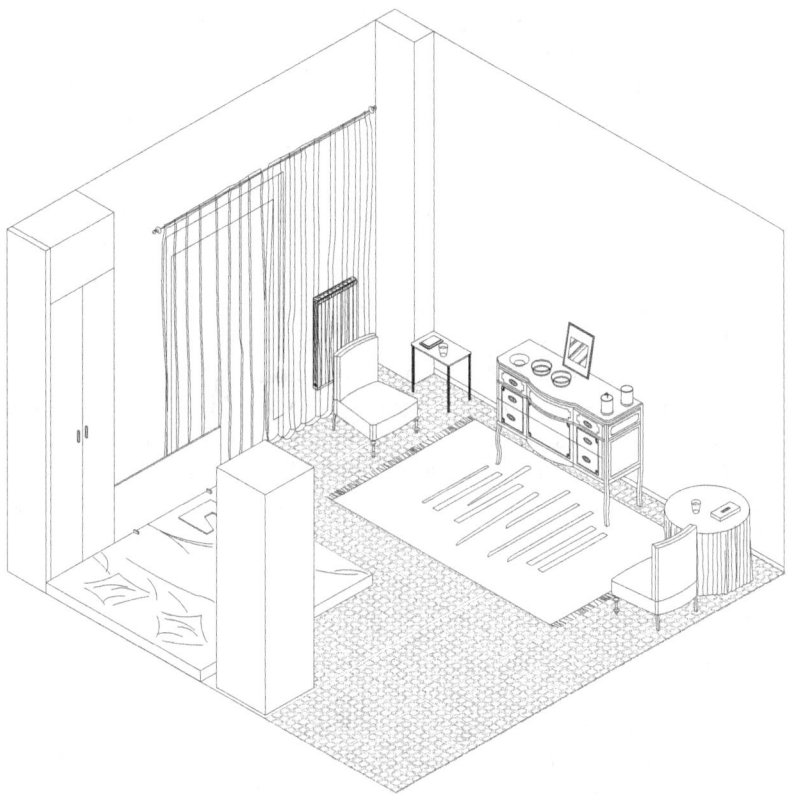

Body psychotherapy, according to Eleni, is a less known modality of psychotherapy. It is based on psychoanalytic and psychodynamic theories and utilises concepts such as the unconscious, transference, defense mechanisms, etc. Its particular emphasis lies in the fact that it focuses on the functional mind–body relationship, considering the complexity of the intersections and interactions between them. All individual approaches of body psychotherapy are based on the core belief that the body reflects personality and that there is a functional unity between mind and body. In body psychotherapy, the term *body* is not identified in its purely biological dimension, and there is no hierarchical relationship between *mind* and *body* or between the *body* and the *psyche*. They are all functional and interacting aspects of the whole of human existence. Body psychotherapy is based on a developmental model, personality theory, hypotheses about the roots of pathogenic symptoms and dysfunctions and a wide range of diagnostic and therapeutic techniques used within the therapy relationship. These techniques include focusing on the body through observation, touch, movement and breathing.[4]

In our first meeting Eleni reports that the room where the sessions are held has a mattress on the floor with some cushions and two armchairs facing each other. She covers all of these with soft fabrics. This is mainly done for practical reasons and not because it 'has to be that way'. She reckons that the ideal space for her work would be a room with three separate zones. A private zone with a desk and a computer, which only the therapist can access, a zone with two armchairs, for the parts of the session that are based on verbal interaction, and a zone with a mattress for the physical part of the therapeutic process. The latter, apart from the mattress and some cushions, should also be equipped with a video projector and a lighting set. Personal items and decorative elements should also be part of the space. Even though the patient is unaware of the history behind these props, Eleni stresses the fact that the presence of the props provides the therapy space with a sense of warmth and intimacy, which is necessary for strengthening the relationship between the therapist and the patient.

Initial ideas

The space is divided into three different parts forming three subsequent subspaces ranging in size, according to the importance of each one of them. The subspaces are the computer room that takes up the smallest share of the whole space, as it plays the least significant role in the therapy process; then, there is the room with the two armchairs facing each other, which occupies a larger area since it is an integral part of the therapy process; and finally, there is the most important room for this particular practice; the room used for physical interaction, which occupies the largest portion of the space due to its major importance and also its prevalent usage in somatic psychotherapy.

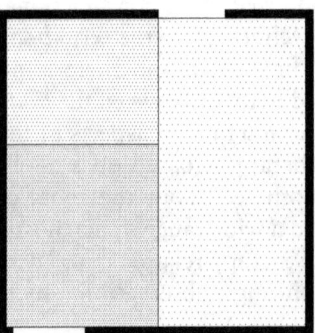
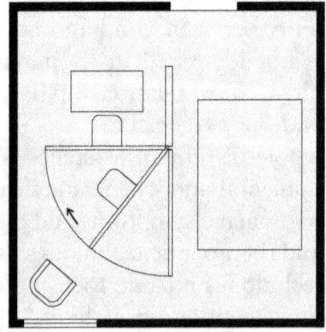

The separation of these spaces is achieved through the use of two partitions. One of the partitions is fixed and is used to divide the original space in two and the other one is modular and placed perpendicularly to the fixed partition. The vertical axis where the two partitions meet is the axis around which the modular partition rotates. The modular partition divides half of the room into two uneven spaces. Both partitions do not extend to the room's surrounding walls, in order to leave enough space for unobstructed peripheral movement. The therapist can move freely in all three spaces, while the patient doesn't have access to the computer room space.

The rotating partition is equipped with a reclining surface. This becomes the therapist's seat. When the therapist is alone, the modular partition is closed, and the seat is reclined towards the computer desk. When there is a patient in the room the modular partition is open, and the seat becomes part of the second space where verbal communication requires seating positions. This moveable seat, apart from saving space, is also used as an element of connection between the two spaces. The main purpose of all the elements used in this first attempt of designing the room is the isolation of each space and the avoidance of interference between different functions.

Presentation of the initial idea/first feedback

In our second meeting, Eleni examined the proposal and mentioned that the idea of this space allocation might prove to be very helpful for the therapy process. She noted that having a private personal space where she could work alone and unobstructed would be very important for her, as it probably would for most therapists. She thought that this structure could really work and that she might try to implement these partitions in the near future. To quote her actual words:

> If I had the opportunity, I would try it. I had thought in the past about putting a screen in the space to achieve the separation of different functions. I didn't. However now, seeing this suggestion, I'm thinking I might give it a try.

However, after examining the proposal for a while, she remarked that she didn't find a strict separation of the two spaces used for therapy really necessary, since they are both used during the time of a typical session. Usually, the process begins with the therapist and the patient entering the room and taking a seat facing each other, then they both move to the mattress area to perform some physical exercises and after that they return to the armchairs for the session to close. The only space that should be isolated is the small computer room. Therefore, she asked if there could be another option where only the computer room would be isolated when the patient is in the space. She stressed that it is important not to only avoid any accidental intrusion, but to also avoid the possibility of visual contact with this space. The boundaries between the space with the armchairs and the space with the mattress could become more discreet or maybe temporary.

Back to the drawing board

After this very helpful feedback the proposal evolved to a more versatile version. The allocation and the size of the subspaces remained, as they were on the first drawing attempt. The fixed partition was cut in half in order to only separate the computer room from the space with the mattress. The modular partition remained as it was but, since half of the fixed partition was removed, it now seems more like a freestanding door.

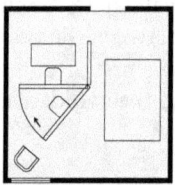 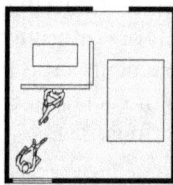 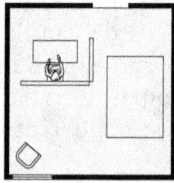 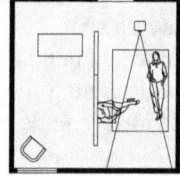

When the therapist is alone, the door can be either open – connecting the computer room to the space with the armchairs – or closed – completely isolating the computer room. When the patient enters the room, the door is closed, and this allows visual and physical connection of the two spaces where the session takes place. The reclining surface that serves as the therapist's chair is still used in this idea. In order to save even more space, but mainly in order to accentuate the flexibility of the design, the reclining surface becomes part of the modular wall. It is produced by a piece of the wall that is cut and can bend up to ninety degrees. According to the placement of the modular wall, the reclining seat could be part of each one of the three separate spaces. This design gesture, however minimal, can easily produce many different versions of the space, totally altering the spatial experience.

Presentation of the process/second feedback

In our final meeting Eleni really appreciated the fact that the space, through the divider, provides her practice with many different possible alternatives. The space is greatly *augmented* and this gives the possibility of another use in some way. She found the proposal really useful, and she was very keen to implement this idea. She also mentioned that the whole process and our meetings gave her many ideas for a future office.

In general, she thought that in therapeutic practice anything that is moving or anything that offers the possibility of multiple uses increases functionality and creates more opportunities. Since most psychotherapists don't have large spaces where they can comfortably do their work, the idea of a structure that changes, conceals, reveals, integrates and isolates different spaces within the same room is a significant opportunity and creates tremendous inspiration for the space of psychotherapy.

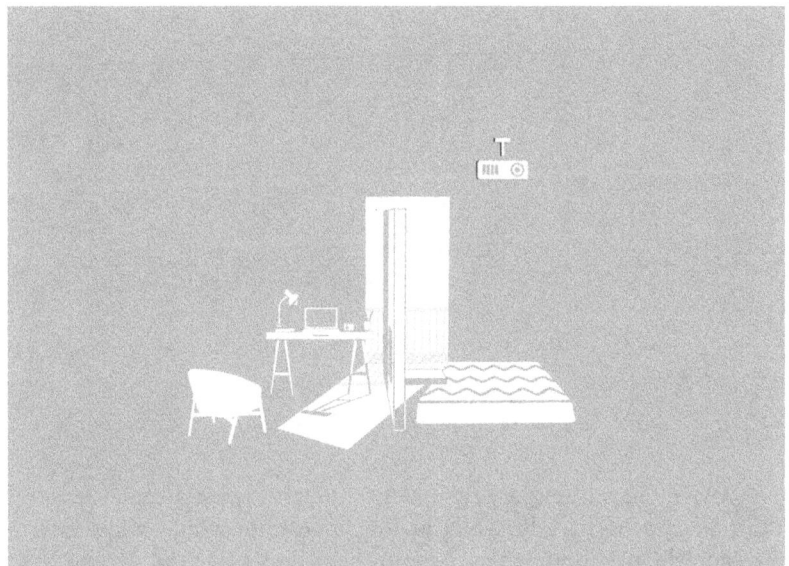

Union

Case study 2: Maria/Ioannina, Greece

The second case study is housed on the ground floor of a typical block of flats located in the historical centre of Ioannina. It is called 'Open Window' and it is self-defined as a *shelter, a place for creative expression*. The therapy practice that is performed within this space is drama therapy. Maria, the owner of the space, notes that the basic principles of drama therapy are related to the use of symbols and metaphors. Progress is made through the healing power of the arts, which, when performed in the right way, can bring the desired evolution and change. Just like the previous example of body psychotherapy, here too the body plays a leading role in the process. Therefore, there is the need for a generous space that provides freedom of movement for a limited number of participants. The room should also accommodate a space for arts and crafts and art materials, i.e., paper, colours and graphic material and also some source of sound. Maria didn't choose the space, but she somehow found herself in it. However, despite the limitations and challenges presented, she managed to create a functional environment for her practice. The space is filled with many vibrant colours that contribute to the artistic atmosphere. On one wall, there is a painting of a tree and a sun. She describes her space as *warm, safe, particular* but also quite *full* in accordance with her full schedule.

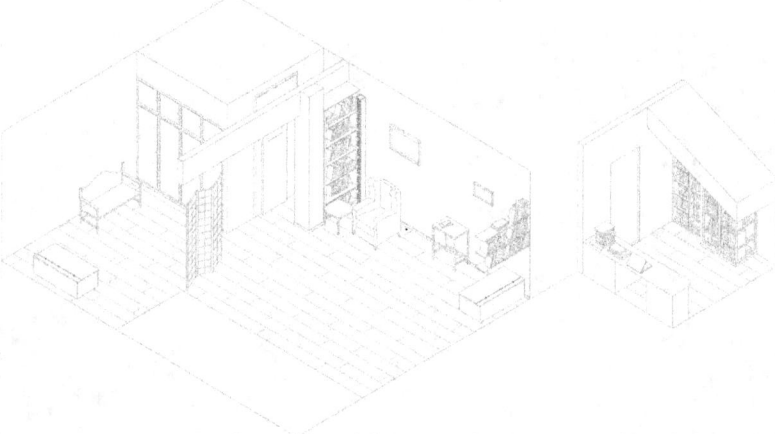

For her, the ideal space would be one that would make her feel that she can be herself, while at the same time would allow her to envision the best potential version of herself. A place that would have strong colours and character. A place that would exude a feeling of life flowing seamlessly. A place filled with the relaxing sounds of the forest.

In conclusion, the elements that seem to have a particular value in this space are nature and the integration of humans in it. The most important factor for the practice of drama therapy seems to be the creation of a transitional space where relationships are mediated through narratives, myths and roleplaying. This takes place in a setting influenced by the natural environment.

Initial ideas

Bearing in mind the particularities of drama therapy, the initial ideas moved within the framework of providing the space with a core element. This element will function as a gathering point. It will act as a point of reference for the group and initiate a centripetal approach.

Because of the therapist's desire to connect with nature this core element could take the form of a tree. In addition to its connection to nature, the tree is also used symbolically. Traditionally in many cultures including the Greek cultural context where this research was conducted, a single tree in a square is the symbol of community. A core element that provides a shelter for meeting and for exchanging ideas. People of all ages share thoughts and feelings, participate in daily social life and very often make important decisions for their place under the shade of a tree.

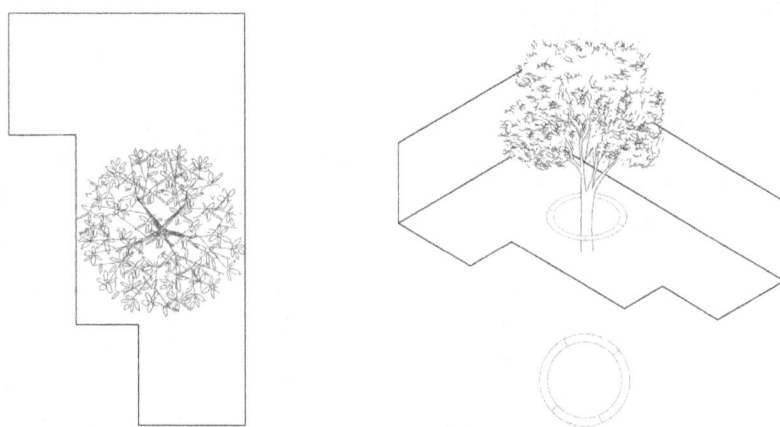

This core element, apart from organising the movement within the space, will also express the notions of balance, harmony, evolution and strength. It will be a *poetic* element that gives a sense of life flowing seamlessly, but it will also inspire a sense of growth and evolution. For this idea to work more efficiently the rest of the space should remain open and unified in order to allow people to interact and feel connected during the group therapy.

Presentation of the initial idea/first feedback

In our second meeting Maria immediately embraced the idea of a natural element. She claimed that she had thought about something similar, several times in the past. Due to lack of space, she had to limit this idea to a two-dimensional mural of a tree. She repeated that if there was enough space, she wouldn't have any second thoughts placing the tree in the space immediately. In her opinion, the tree fits in very well on a symbolic level as well. It is a very intense stimulus that would help the process of drama therapy. Placing it in a central point could also prove very effective for eliminating the awkwardness of an empty space. The ideas of balance and harmony that were mentioned previously also seemed very important, especially since we are dealing with a space where therapy takes place. Maria is very keen to see the progress of this idea in our next meeting.

Back to the drawing board

The first discussion proved very helpful, as there was a consensus on the importance of a design element that would evoke nature. After some time on the drawing board and a number of sketches on the initial plan, the idea of the tree evolved into an abstract representation of it. An organic sculptural structure that touches the ground and becomes bigger and wider as it approaches the space's ceiling. A shape that doesn't imitate the form of a tree but tries to capture the essence of growth and evolution instead. The form was placed in the centre of the main space. This gesture strengthened the concept of gathering that we were contemplating. However, it seemed isolated and a bit too self-referential. Therefore, it started to become clear that this central form could be the beginning of a more generous design approach.

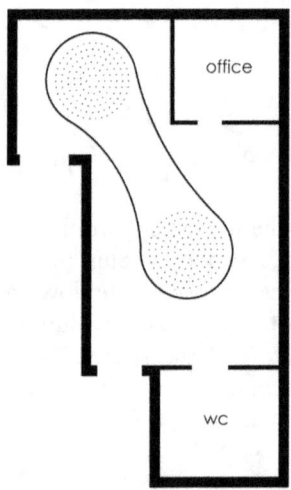
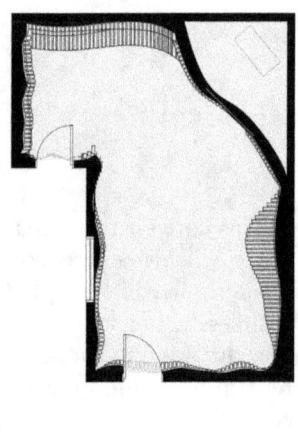

The form was analysed into curved contours made of wood. This design technique is easy to implement onto any surface. Therefore, the contours took over the walls and became seating spaces and a second tree-like form was designed in the rear end of the room. The implementation of a single design gesture in the whole space gave a sense of flow and union. The two treelike structures differ in materiality. The bigger one in the centre of the room is hard and rigid and the smaller one, which is proposed to be made by the repetition of elastic strips, is soft and more flexible.

The general vibe that the room now exudes is one of harmony and flow. The space allows for the development of several different scenarios and functions. It encourages creative thinking and perception as well as the development of imagination.

Presentation of the process/second feedback

Maria was surprised to see how this idea evolved but quite soon she was drawn to the idea of an organic structure taking over the whole space. She reckoned that the spaces could now have so many uses. The treelike structures stand as both boundaries and scenographic elements contributing to the therapeutic process. The walls that become an augmented seating space seem like a very elegant and space-saving idea.

Although this new idea seemed a bit eccentric and challenging to construct, Maria was really keen on trying it at some point. She thought that the proposed space could play a more active role in the drama therapy process. From our point of view, the most important part of this second meeting was that Maria said that our dialogues helped her realise what a difference it makes to let the ideas evolve and take shape through the discussion with a designer. She found this process both creative and impactful and it inspired her to open up to this new world of ideas.

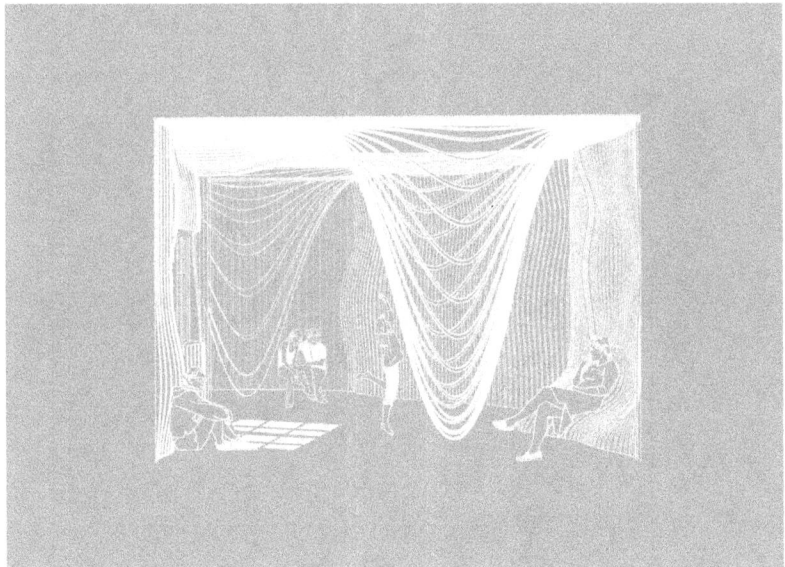

Immersion

Case study 3: Charlotte/London, U.K.

The third case study is Charlotte's space. Charlotte is a psychotherapist based in Northwest London. She practises psychoanalytic psychotherapy from a relational perspective. She states that the basic principle of psychoanalytic psychotherapy is the connection between the past and the present, which is expressed through free association.

The patterns that recur in the narrative and in the life of the analysand mirror this connection between the past and the present.

It is important for the psychoanalytic space to encourage free association and to harbour the therapy relationship between the analyst and the analysand. Some of the elements that encourage this free association within the context of the therapy process are armchairs at an angle from each other, the psychoanalytic couch, low lighting, quietness, colour as well as a selection of artwork.

Her consulting room is housed in her home. She reckons that, in her opinion, psychoanalytic work is built in the liminal space of the threshold between the personal and the professional. In a sense, this could be the therapist's personal space, where she welcomes and makes room for her patients' free associations.

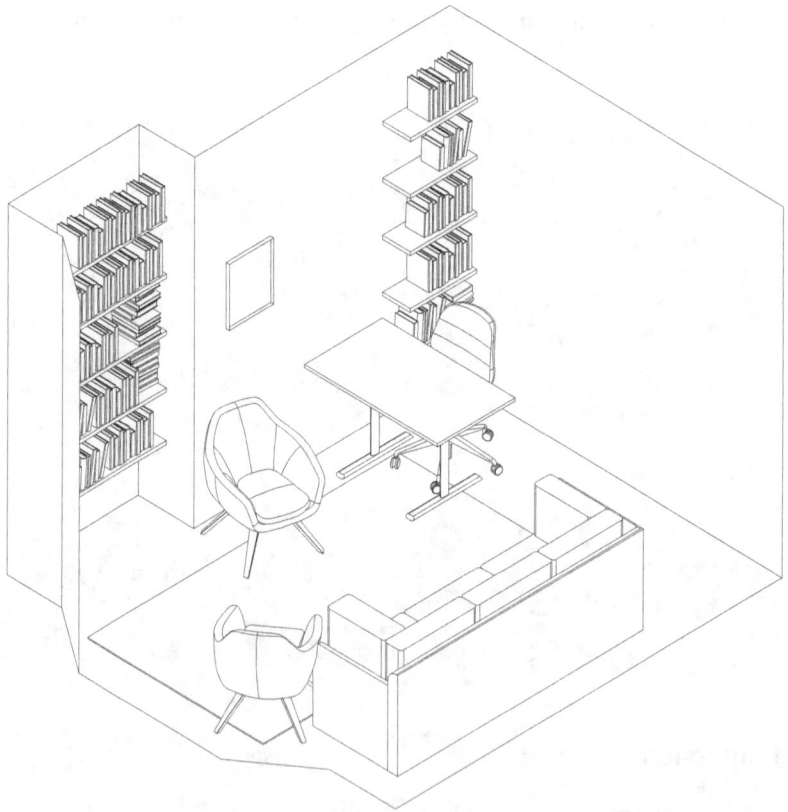

She noted that she always felt that if she, as a therapist, was not in an organic and personal relationship with the space where she practised psychotherapy, it would have a negative effect on her ability to help her patients get in touch with deep emotions and the unconscious.

There must be an opportunity for rapport for both members of the therapeutic relationship.

Elements such as cultural diversity, hybridity and the complexity of human relationships are important in her practice and she would like her office to reflect this. There are always plants in her space, which she believes symbolise life and the growth of the therapy relationship.

In her ideal office, the style would be similar to her current office, quite contemporary and urban with quirky personal touches. A space with bright colours and bold style combinations that would facilitate the existence of otherness.

For this case, our design approach will revolve around finding a way in which the analysand could enter into a state of immersion into their inner process. We will try to propose an environment that will encourage free association within the context of the therapy relationship.

Initial ideas

Taking as a central axis some core concepts of psychoanalytic psychotherapy such as free association and repetitive patterns and keeping the exact square meters and shape of the space in mind, the idea is formulated as follows. First a grid of cubes is placed on the ground. The dimensions of the cubes can hypothetically allow one to sit or lie down. Subsequently, the cubes are extruded to different heights and form prisms of different dimensions (0.5 m, 0.8 m, 1.1 m). The cubes are made of soft foamy material, in order to provide comfort for both the therapist and the patient. A similar pattern of cubes is placed on the ceiling. The hanging cubes function as storage space, shelves and bookcases.

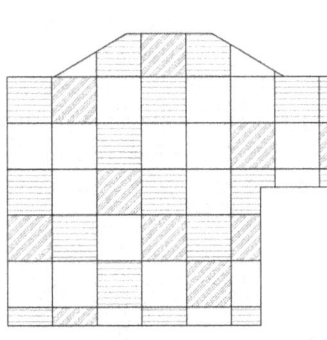
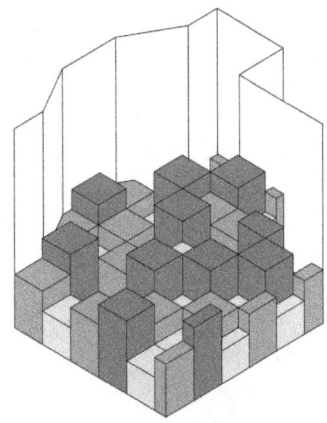

When the patient enters the space, they are presented with different options of interacting with it. They can sit or lie down in a number of different positions. They are presented with various alternatives they can use depending on their moods. The general idea is immersion, a dive into the unconscious, the inner self. Therefore, the design concept, besides being flexible and functional, also becomes symbolic. The uneven adventurous *floor* becomes the means that allows the notions of complexity and otherness, discussed in our first meeting, to manifest themselves.

Presentation of the initial idea/first feedback

In our second meeting, Charlotte was enthusiastic about this idea. She found it very imaginative and noticed that the concept is a precise translation of her answers in the questionnaire given to her in advance. She said that she would love her space to allow for so many different possibilities and that she believes that besides its unconventional layout, the space could be very helpful for her work and the process of psychotherapy.

In her feedback, Charlotte asked if we could consider the idea of one or two prisms taking up the whole height of the room and maybe acquiring another function. She also mentioned that, although she understands why the space is filled with prisms, she would like to see a few gaps between them that would facilitate movement.

Finally, she noted that the concept of immersion is core in her way of practising psychotherapy, and she was happily surprised to see how this concept can be translated into space. She was also very impressed by the expressive ability she saw in the first sketches.

Back to the drawing board

After this particularly constructive discussion, the proposal is formulated as follows: the grid is maintained, but the cubes on the floor are raised to different heights. Some places on the gird remain empty, forming a passage from one part of the room to another. The cubes are arranged in a sort of amphitheatrical way so that there is no visual barrier between the therapist and the patient. One of the prisms extends up to the ceiling and has multiple uses. It is used as a bookcase and also as a backrest for two sides of the seats. The number of reclining positions has also increased.

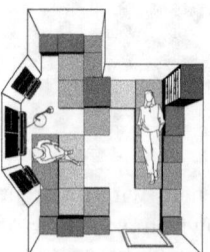 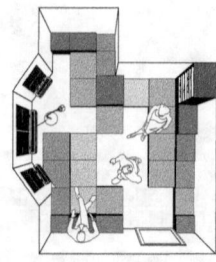 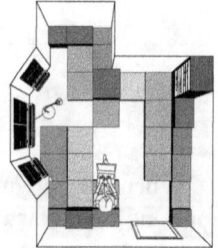

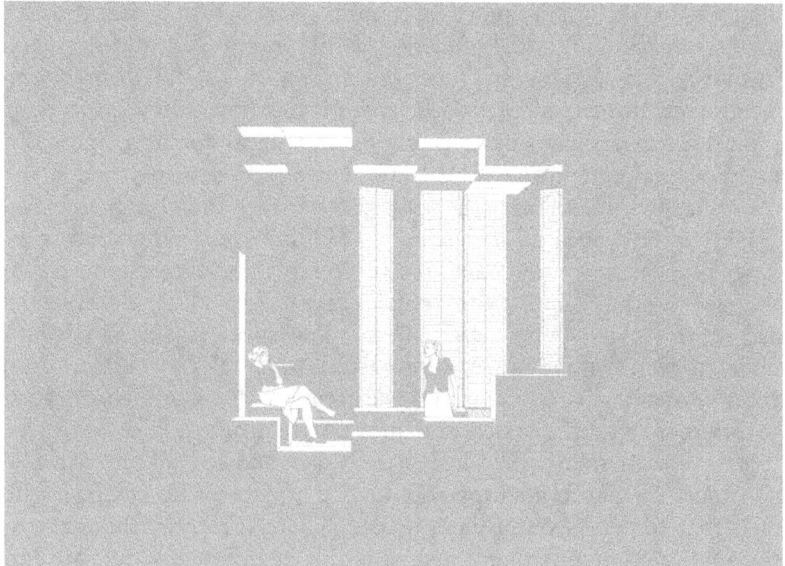

A matching complementary pattern of prisms is placed on the ceiling. These can become storage places and dimmable lighting fixtures. The space can be used both during psychotherapy and for the therapist's personal work.

Presentation of the process/second feedback

In our final meeting Charlotte was really happy to see the results. She found the final design wonderful and claimed that she would really consider implementing it. She called the space *a playroom*, an interesting idea that captures well the way that she works.

Her feedback was that that our discussion allowed for an accurate translation of the way she described her practice. She thought that the drawings were perceptive and accurate and that the whole process exuded creative energy that left her with a desire to seriously think of taking the risk of changing her space.

Reflection

Case 4: Sasha/Scotland

The fourth case study is a consulting room in Scotland belonging to Sasha. Sasha practices transactional and psychodynamic psychotherapy. Her therapy approach is based on existential philosophy, psychoanalytic anthropology and psychotherapy applied to culturally transformative phenomena, such as child-rearing practices that shape adult personality. In her practice, cultural symbols that appear through myths, dreams and rituals function as parables or allegories of performance. Interactions are interpreted using analytical theories and techniques. In her practice, Sasha investigates how social institutions raise defense mechanisms or create psychological conflicts. She has a particular interest in the cross-cultural application of psychoanalytic concepts, such as exploring the space between race and phenomenology.

Her office is located in her home. She believes that the environment plays a very important role in therapy, and this is reflected in the way she has shaped the 'setting' in which it takes place. There are several places where one can sit. The space is decorated with many objects belonging to different cultures. It is a multicultural, creative space where people can feel intimate. Users are encouraged to interact with the space and move the furniture. They are free to create their own world inside the space and let her enter it. She considers the psychotherapy room to be a place of negotiation. She feels that sometimes as a therapist she has to surrender the space to the analysand and let them shape it in the way that they feel safe and comfortable, and which allows them to communicate more effectively (Danze, 2005).

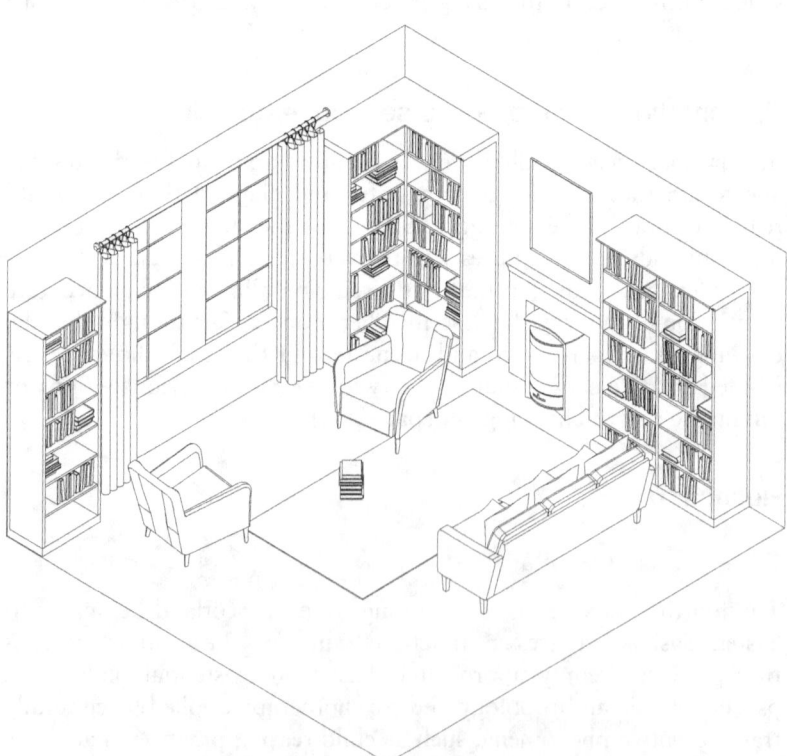

The ideal space for her would be Sigmund Freud's consulting room. Therefore, she tried to recreate this atmosphere (Fuss & Sanders, 2004). She decorated her consulting room with Persian rugs, bold colors, fabrics and heavy furniture (Engelman, 1981).

In an effort to translate her method of work, the design approach is centered around the idea of creating a room where both the analyst and the analysand would have a comfortable experience, without interfering with each other's perception of the space. It is important for the two personalities to fit simultaneously in the same space without having direct contact, until the moment that they decide to start the interaction.

Initial ideas

The main concept revolves around the separation of space into two sections. The space for the analyst and the space for the analysand. Both spaces are well defined. The analysand has the freedom to reconfigure almost the entire section of their space, until they find a place where they can feel safe and ready to initiate the interaction with the therapist. The fact that the room already has two different entrances facilitates this concept.

Somewhere in the middle of the room there will be a divider that can open and close. When the patient enters the room, the divider will be closed allowing no visual contact with the space allocated to the therapist. Patients are able to reconfigure the space as they wish and when they feel ready and find a suitable place, they can open the divider, so that the session can begin. When the therapist is alone in the space for personal work, the divider can remain open.

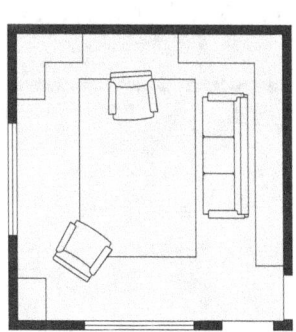 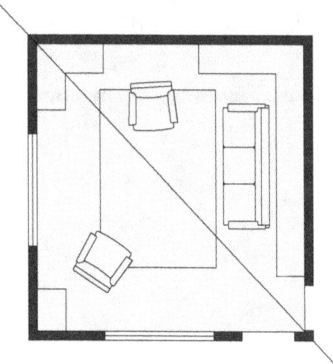

The proposal aims to partially isolate each space and to unite it when the patient feels comfortable enough to begin the interaction with the therapist. The idea of mirroring is related to two different characteristics of the space. Primarily it is referring to the creation of two almost identical spaces facing each other. On a deeper level, it reflects the therapist's ambition and her wish to recreate the archetypal space of psychotherapy, which is Freud's office in Bergasse Street, which is still an important reference for many consulting rooms around the world (see Gerald, 2020).

Presentation of the initial idea/first feedback

In our second meeting, Sasha was intrigued by the concept of dividing and reuniting the space. She thought that it accurately captured and translated the dynamics of her therapeutic approach and encaptulated the notions of creation, form, revelation and concealment. In her opinion, it is very important how people frame the idea of space in their minds. She reckons that the psychotherapy consulting room is a metaphorical space and that she finds the way this is conceptualised through design very effective. She also believes that working in this environment could be both functional and comfortable.

Back to the drawing board

The next step of the design process is defining the position, the form and the materiality of the partition. To facilitate entrance from both sides of the space and to eliminate any encounter prior to the beginning of the therapy process, it is placed diagonally in the room creating two spaces of triangular shape. In order for the partition to be light and easily moveable, it is made out of vertical blinds. Each one of the blinds also has the ability to rotate around its axis, giving the opportunity for several scenarios of openness and closeness. They can be pulled to one side to completely unite the room or rotate in different angles to allow different degrees of visibility between the two spaces.

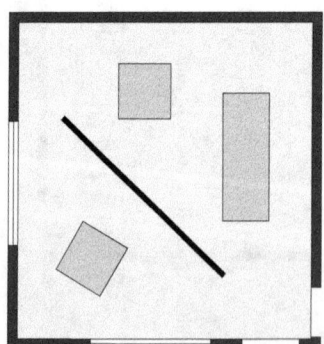 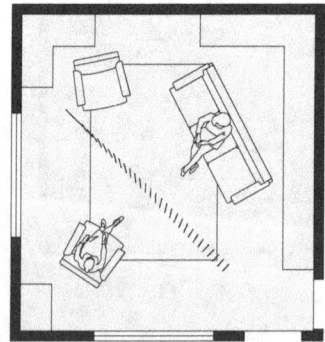

When the analysand enters their part of the consulting room, the therapist is in her place and the vertical blinds closed. There is no eye contact between the two. On the part allocated to the analysand, there are several versions of reconfiguring the space. If they choose, they can lie down, sit in the armchair or even on the floor. They can also move the furniture, if they find that this is what they need to do in order to make themselves feel comfortable. Once the analysand has configured the space and they feel ready to begin therapy, they reveal themselves as much as they feel comfortable by opening the partition to the degree they judge appropriate.

On the side of the analysand there is of course the psychoanalytic couch, an armchair and some of the bookcases. Similarly on the therapist's side there is her armchair and some bookcases. To accentuate the notion of reflection, the vertical blinds are covered by a semi-reflective material. The mirror-like surface creates on a perception level the impression of completing the space through duplication. On a symbolic level, it is used to show that even when divided the space can be perceived as a whole. On a second symbolic level, it is used to reference Freud's office where mirrors played a significant part in the arrangement of the space (Schroeder, 2020).

Presentation of the process/second feedback

Sasha was once again enthusiastic about the evolution of the project. She mentioned that concealment and disclosure are very closely related to the conscious self and the unconscious. She thought that the proposal expressed a dynamic that feels right in the context of analytic therapy. She explained that in psychoanalysis fragments are a big part of the process (Fuss, 2004). Therefore, when the blinds are partially open and rotating, the image one faces is broken into fragments. When they are fully opened the pieces of the image come together and we are witnessing something complete.

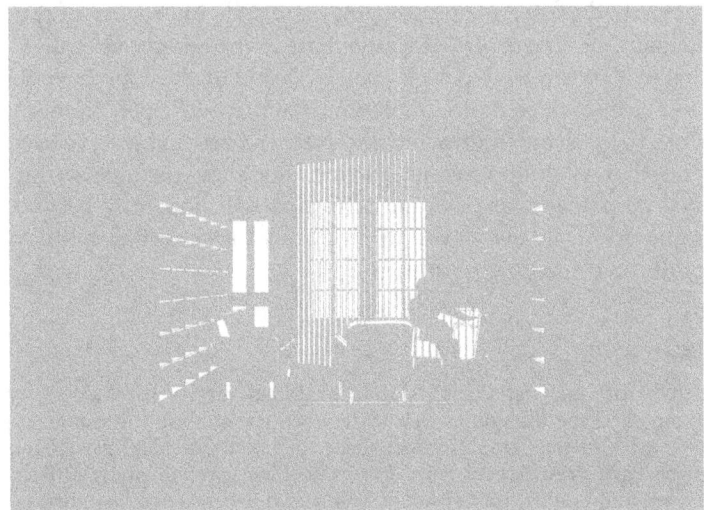

Conclusion

An important axiom of this research from the beginning of its conception was that we wouldn't resolve to stereotypes and preconceived ideas about the space of psychotherapy consulting rooms. Instead, it would be open to the unforeseen and we would let ideas evolve organically through discussion and feedback. Luckily, the four therapists that took part in this process were open enough to allow space for experimentation and play. Each one of the proposals is unique and it is centered around the four therapists' views and aspirations and their ways of expressing them. However, even if each proposal is custom designed to fit into a specific consulting room, the process and the methodology applied could be implemented in several other cases of therapy spaces. Experimenting with the ideas of transition, union, immersion and reflection is not new to architects and designers. All of the design strategies that were applied, however imaginative or even quirky, are standard in architectural projects. The innovation lies in the fact that it is not common to consider these ideas as suitable for spaces where therapy takes place, which apparently remain very faithful to their archetypal forms.

The research methodology was inspired by the therapy process, which is based on the one-on-one relationship and dialogue, as well as the therapist's ability for careful listening. In our case, the dialogue was initiated between the therapist and the designer. The aim of the project was to find a unique spatial configuration that can encourage the therapy process in these four different modalities of psychotherapy as they were perceived, presented and practiced by each individual practitioner. An even more important aim was to test if this spatial configuration could be achieved through a method of discussion, namely dialogue and feedback facilitated by drawings, images and sketches. As mentioned earlier, the personalities and style of practice of the four participant therapists played a large part in the design process.

This is a research by design project. None of the four case studies reached a final degree of completion. They are all open to more discussion, more detailed drawing and further fine-tuning. However, the process that all four research participants went through so far has opened up a world of possibilities, which will hopefully become the springboard for a new way of approaching the sensitive, multilayered space of the consulting room.

Notes

1 Even before the pandemic, Mark Gerald addresses the issue of online sessions and the difficulties that arise when the analyst and the analysand don't meet in the same physical space. In his article 'The Psychoanalytic Office: Past, Present, and Future' (Gerald, The Psychoanalytic Office: Past Present, and Future, 2011) he writes: 'It is not necessary to be in one's office

to conduct a session on the phone or by computer. How do we belong as psychoanalysts, if our offices with their collections of belongings cease to be our exclusive place of work? The usual objects that are associated with our defining sense of ourselves are not always present if we work from locations that are remote from our offices'.
2 Most of this evidence can be found in the photographic work of Engelman (Engelman, 1981).
3 All names of participants are pseudonyms to preserve confidentiality. Written consent has been granted from all of them.
4 More information can be found on the following website by the Greek Association of Body Psychotherapy: www.pesops.gr/zzz/pesops.php (Greek Association for Body Psychotherapy, 2022).

References

Danze, E. (2005). An architects view of introspective space: The analytic vessel. *Annual of Psychoanalysis, 33*, 109–124.

Engelman, E. (1981). *Berggasse 19: Sigmund Freud's home and offices, Vienna, 1938: The photographs of Edmund Engelman.* University of Chicago Press.

Fuss, D. (2004). *The sense of an interior: Four writers and the rooms that shaped them.* Routledge.

Fuss, D., & Sanders, J. (2004). Freud's ear: Bergasse 19 Vienna Austria. In D. Fuss (Ed.), *The sense of an interior: Four writers and the rooms that shaped them* (p. 75). Routledge.

Gerald, M. (2020). *In the shadow of Freud's couch: Portraits of psychoanalysts and their offices.* Routledge.

Greek Association for Body Psychotherapy. (2022, November 10). Retrieved Greek Association for Body Psychotherapy: www.pesops.gr/zzz/pesops.php

Schroeder, J. K. (2020). The active room: Freud's office and the Egyptian tomb. *Frontiers in Psychology.* https://doi.org/10.3389/fpsyg.2020.01547.

Part 3

The online consulting room during the COVID-19 pandemic and beyond

8   The screen therapy room
Real flowers in a digital vase
Dora Tsogia

Introduction

Having inspected the therapy room for one last time, I couldn't help feeling a sense of excitement for what was about to happen. Finally, I was going to meet a patient in person. It felt so long that I couldn't remember when I had seen her last, not on screen, which was weekly, but in the 'real', three dimensions, occupying space, sat in my blue armchair, resting her feet on the carpet, fiddling with her bag, generally 'sensing someone'. I imagined hearing the bell, my patient walking through the garden, ringing the bell. I looked at my watch, realising I had another few minutes left, so I inspected the hallway entrance once again, which on that particular day seemed to be taking part in the revival of my consulting room too, having been unnoticed for weeks on end. I put my mask on, waiting for my patient to arrive, and as I was rearranging the fresh yellow flowers in the vase near the entrance, my eye caught my mobile's light going on. 'Dr. Tsogia, can we have the session on skype again? I am feeling a bit under the weather, so just to be on the safe side . . .' What a disappointment. Of course, it was to be on the safe side, but still . . . As I prepared my laptop for the session, I decided not to take my smart shoes off as I usually did, choosing the comfort of my sneakers. I would conduct the session as if my patient was really there, plants watered, shoes on. Fifty minutes later, as I was closing the lid of my laptop, I took another decision: from now on, my vase would never be empty again. I would keep buying those nice flowers for my vase at the entrance, as a welcoming gesture, as I always used to. (Perhaps I could keep my sneakers on, they didn't seem to make a difference.)

When was it that having sessions online became our normality? Is it as effective? Does it actually *feel* the same? What happens to our senses during an online session? Did we ever wonder what happens to our senses within the therapy room in the first place? How is vision, sound, smell, taste or touch affected in therapy? How can I use them now? After a few years of on-and-off lockdowns now, we have certainly learnt a few things. For one, the fact that we must not take anything for granted in that psychotherapy space, but instead, reflect carefully on what it is we have to offer and how therapy online changes the way

DOI: 10.4324/9781003346845-12

we work. No therapist must enter this new situation lightheartedly. I remember watching my kids doing martial arts online, during the first lockdown. The emotions I experienced were a mixture of sadness and joy: sad for all they were missing, joyful for attempting to find a solution, not giving up. Is this what we, therapists and patients and trainees and supervisors, are doing? Not giving up? And, perhaps more importantly, does online therapy feel the same as in-person therapy? And is it effective? No, it doesn't always feel exactly the same. Yes, I believe it can be as effective. Perhaps not for all (patients), perhaps not by all (therapists). It all depends on how one perceives, approaches and processes the whole matter. In the present chapter, I will be sharing my thoughts about my experience of online therapy, informed by some relevant literature. By no means is this meant to be an extensive review of the literature or a debate about the pros and cons of online therapy, but rather a reflection through clinical experience.

Beginnings

'Hello? I can't see you. Can you see me?' 'Can you hear me?'
'Oh wait, I must plug this in, the battery is very low.'
'Is the light ok? Is it too dark?'

These are some of the first words a therapist often hears on screen. How different this is from the ordinary opening of a therapy session, ranging from the awkward mentioning of the weather or the traffic from some to the immediate mentioning of a dream or a continuation of what was being explored at the end of the last session.

N.,[1] a forty-five-year-old woman suffering from health anxiety and long-term depression, was previously coming to my office, always commenting on the style and decoration. She liked the colors in the room and felt very comfortable in her seat. In the aftermath of two years of lockdowns, N. has not been able to travel to my therapy room, too frightened to use public transport. The external world has become persecutory for her more than ever. The beginning of our online sessions is always in relation to the poor sound of her laptop, as if she does not need to change that, reflecting perhaps some inner sense of being isolated from the rest of the world in order to be protected. She then comments on the colors of my consulting room that she can see in the background and how much she misses being there. When she previously came to sessions in person, she would also have a 'ritual' in the beginning, complaining about people in the underground and how they behaved. The new routine seems to have replaced the previous one, with an opening line often being something like 'oh that blue armchair'!

In the same way that someone enters a therapy room according to their character and issues, they also enter an 'online therapy room' in a specific manner each time, thinking about practicalities or diving into the subject matter.

Mask vs screen

One of the things I have missed most in my practice during the last few years when I see patients in the room is seeing a person's full face. Wearing masks in the consulting room is customary in in-person therapy in Greece, even after the end of lockdowns. There is the occasional taking off the mask, if someone is too upset or has difficulty breathing, but as a general rule we both keep our masks on. If I was asked whether I prefer to continue working one way or the other, I would probably opt for seeing the whole face, even online. Facial expressions, smiling or not, can give much more away than someone's physical presence!

The two words, both of medieval origin (mask appearing for the first time in English in the 1530s, deriving from medieval Latin), and screen (of more uncertain origin, though probably from a Germanic source, perhaps from Middle Dutch according to Wiktionary) are used with a similar meaning: *mask* means 'to hide or protect the face', whereas *screen* also refers to a 'physical object of protection'. The way the words are used, however, indicates an important difference: mask implies hiding, not showing parts of the face; whereas the word screen is more associated with protecting and filtering through. The question is, how much is filtered through in screen therapy that perhaps should not be? What happens to our senses when we are conducting psychotherapy online?

What happens to our senses?

My therapist's consulting room was roughly a half-hour drive from my place. A long road connecting my unconscious with someone else's, that's how it felt driving there in the early morning. When the traffic was not bad it took half the time, and then I would go to the corner coffee house by Moseley Road, have a cup of tea, just gathering my thoughts before my session. Is it time? I would walk to my therapist's practice, enter the nicely kept garden. There I am, ringing the bell. There he is, same posture each time, opening the door, greeting me with a slight smile. The discreet, but present odour of the house would hit my nostrils, my eye would catch yellow or white flowers in some vase . . . The blue cover on the couch, a nod to begin.

This is how I remember getting to my own psychotherapy many years back, smells and colours involved. Perhaps an unfair comparison to make with an online session, with someone preparing their own space, perhaps their own tea, tidying up their background, pressing the Zoom or Skype button. The senses are still involved, even if there is less element of surprise. What invisible route is now connecting one's unconscious with someone else's when they get ready for their online session? Having a ritual to enter one's psychotherapy is what remains constant and may involve various senses. I have heard of both patients and therapists burning incense and preparing teas and putting on their favorite covers . . . We cannot argue it is the same, what I am arguing however is that the senses are involved in both situations. In the case of online therapy, however, the therapist has no effect on the sensory input to their patients other than the visual and auditory ones, and those are also subject to transmission problems that may arise during the session.

Do you mind me staring at you?

Where should one look at during an online session? In our training, we had learnt that eye contact is vital, but that at the same time it should not feel threatening, that is you should not make the patient feel they are being stared at. Balancing this comes naturally when meeting someone face to face, based on one's social skills too. But using a screen makes a difference. The other person cannot actually see where you are looking, when you are not looking at them. Some writers suggest it is less intense (Anastasopoulos, 2017), but I found it to be the opposite. It is a common experience how freeing the use of couch is on those matters. I recall a certain session during lockdown, which was conducted with the camera off, because of a technical problem, and how my patient eventually said how this enabled her to speak more freely. She even considered starting to use the couch when the lockdown ended. Eventually, I have resorted to not looking at the screen constantly for the whole fifty minutes, in the same way that I wouldn't be staring at someone constantly in the room for fifty minutes! When we think, our eyes wander a little anyway, so I thought this came as a natural process. In one session, however, I realised this may not be how patients perceive this change.

> In one of those moments when I was resting my gaze on the carpet, thinking about what was being said, N. (mentioned previously) said to me, obviously irritated, 'Do you want to finish whatever it is you are doing first?' I realised she thought I was looking at my mobile or something else, which proved useful material to think about, but also highlighted the potential difficulty in the therapy relationship when a big part of our physical environment during the session is hidden from the patient.

Seeing too much

We cannot ignore serious voices that tell us to be careful about the use of technology in therapy, such as Russell's (2015). Amongst other issues, Russell suggests that the therapist sees too much from the patient's personal environment, which is not what happens in traditional therapy. Despite the numerous times a patient may tell us 'you'd have to be there to understand', we know it's best not to 'be there', and that the psychoanalytic work takes place in the microcosm that therapist and patient build together, in a safe place. A cat walking across the keyboard, an unmade bed in the background, the particular posters or paintings a patient chooses to put on their wall are only examples of information one would not have had it been a face-to-face session in the therapist's consulting room. However, one could argue that this is not necessarily a negative thing. Psychoanalytic thinking also suggests that the patient will give to the therapist the fragments of their world that they need the therapist to contain and process at a certain time. The extra information given 'accidentally', however, can be seen as a slip of attention the same as other Freudian slips, and can be used productively in the therapy work.

> S., a woman in her early 30s, a musician, had moved abroad after two years of in-person therapy. We continued working online, and even though she had had this experience of the stable and safe space of the consulting room for two years, she kept changing her location in the house during online therapy. In one session, she said that she was too ill to get out of bed, but did not want to cancel the therapy that day. She sat up in bed and we carried on with the session, not realising, as she said later, that the bigger part of my screen would have been covered by a painting she had over her bed, the 'Origins of the world', by Goustave Courbet[2] (L'Origine du monde – Gustave Courbet | Musée d'Orsay (musee-orsay.fr)). For those familiar with the painting, it is obvious it was not an easy subject to raise. When I did though, uncomfortable as it may have been, it proved to be a useful accidental 'slip' of her attention as to which parts of her life she wanted me to see, and what that painting meant to her. The most suitable interpretation that came to mind in this case was that she wanted to focus more on issues of sexuality in her therapy, but couldn't bring herself to articulate this. She accepted the interpretation with a sense of relief. In this case, we managed to take a useful path we might not have taken otherwise, but I can understand that not all patients would be ready to do this kind of work, and in this case interpreting the symbolism in their background would only be felt as an interruption.

I found reading other therapists' similar experiences very comforting at the time, as this was a new situation. Like Gutierrez (2017), I found myself feeling trapped in the screen of my laptop, being moved from room to room, and even knowing I am in the private space of my patient and being forced to face the painting over her bed.

Another point of interest is that, as Skleidi (2017) suggests, the therapist's and patient's faces on screen are closer than they would ever be in the therapy room, causing intense and complex emotions. The 'safe distance', carefully balanced in the therapy consulting room, is abolished, and an experience of an unnatural closeness takes its place. Except for bearing this in mind and reflecting upon its possible effects, we have the responsibility to use our clinical judgement as to who can bear such 'closeness' and who can't. As with psychoanalytic work in general, online therapy, whatever the approach, may not be suitable for everyone. Anastasopoulos (2017) offers some rough guidelines regarding possible indications and contraindications when considering suitability for online therapy.[3]

Silence on the screen

Winnicott drew our attention to the situation where one is alone in the presence of the other, 'the capacity to be alone', a capacity based on the early experience of a good internal object (Winnicott, 1958). Silence in a session can be experienced as such a moment, where productive but separate being and thinking can take place, when this capacity is in place, or as a persecutory one, when it isn't. There are different qualities of silence in a session (Gutierrez, 2107), and the screen poses an extra challenge. In my experience, silence is the most affected condition in online therapy, reminding me of my trainee years, when silence would be felt like an awkward social situation rather than a necessary safe space for both participants in order to think. Similarly to other therapists (Russell, 2015; Anastasopoulos, 2017), I initially found it very hard to maintain silent moments online, perhaps due to the uncertainty that it *was* a silent moment and the screen had not just frozen due to a bad connection. It takes some time to get used to this, but often one of the two participants breaks the silent moment asking 'can you hear me?' Despite the fact that supporters of online therapy believe that even such moments can bring transference issues to the focus that can be then worked with, I find that the silent moments have diminished in my online sessions.

Do I smell cake?

Entering someone else's home or practice always involves sensing the particular building's odour, whether discreet or not. This is something that is definitely missed in online sessions. The sense of smell however cannot be shared by the two parties of the therapeutic dyad, but carries on as usual for each of them. Familiar odors, those of one's own house, office, etc., may enter the therapeutic space.

> Our online session with K. was about halfway through, when she sniffed the air, as if sensing something odd. My immediate thoughts concerned her safety, where what actually happened was that getting 'lost', in a way, within our therapeutic space, she forgot she had to take a cake out of the oven at a certain time. Of course, then the question arose: why put a cake in the oven when she knew she had to go into her session? Having difficulties with boundaries, she got carried away trying to 'fit' her therapy around her household. She solved the issue by opening a door and asking someone else to take the cake out of the oven for her. The door closed again, but chores, husbands, odours had already intruded into our session.

Smoke on the screen

It is not an uncommon occasion in Greece for the public transport workers, among others, to be on strike. On one of those occasions recently, I had my first online session with B., a sixty-year-old woman who was in therapy with me for a few months. Relieved to see our full faces for the first time, B. said that an online session wasn't so bad after all, smiled, sipped her coffee and said that she felt privileged to be able to smoke her electronic cigarette during our session as well. The screen was soon filled with smoke, herself happily set in the comfort of her own environment.

The stricter psychoanalytic part of my training made me worry when this occurred. I tried to see it from a broader perspective, but my thoughts were along the lines of, 'What is she doing here? Can this be useful therapy material? Is the smoke directed at me or does it reflect a fog in her mind?' In a similar manner as mentioned earlier regarding the matter of silence, all such issues can be useful to work with. This proved to be a very productive session, focusing on matters that B. usually had difficulty talking about. Could it have been the unveiling of masks? Or was it the comfort of her home and smoking her cigarette?

Some writers suggest that there is evidence that patients express themselves more easily online on intimate subjects, perhaps due to the object (laptop) being treated as an extension of the self and cyberspace part of one's psychic world (Gutierrez, 2017). Suler (2004) calls it the 'online disinhibition effect'. But what about boundaries? Should I have asked her to treat the invisible therapy room as if it were real, therefore not smoking or having her coffee? Following my therapeutic intuition, I did not intervene, which proved to be right in this case. The 'fog' influenced my reverie in this session, wondering what she does not want me to see, or even at certain moments, whether the blowing the smoke towards the screen felt aggressive towards me. Dilemmas like this often arise during online sessions, as they do during in-person sessions. Whether a therapist 'allows' the patient to sip their tea, or to have a tea themselves, all goes back to their training, experience and clinical judgement as to what will be more productive and appropriate in each case. As Skleidi (2017) stresses, a therapist's adequacy to work online also depends on their willingness and openness to reflect on such matters and on the changes online therapy brings to the process of therapy.

Say hi to the doctor

Another session with K.: the door opened again, her two-year-old had slipped away from his carer's attention, he was crying for his mummy. After taking him on her lap, K. told him to 'say hi to the doctor'. He looked at me between his tears, waiting perhaps for the usual 'baby' talk adults do with infants, and there I was, face-to-face on screen with a cute toddler, trying to maintain a therapeutic stance . . .

Obvious as it is that K. has issues with maintaining boundaries, this vignette shows how vital it is to clarify the therapy framework before starting online sessions, even if it is a continuation of a therapy that was taking place in person before. This incident occurred early on in my 'online' experience – not that it cannot happen now. But as long as the therapist has set out the therapy framework, she makes it easier for the patient not to get confused and for example forget to lock doors or bake cakes during a session. However, as Gutierrez (2017) points out, for some patients online therapy entails the risk of promoting a forced ego integration, as the sometimes necessary 'regression to dependency' (Winnicott, 1955) is not entirely feasible online. The responsibility to protect their own space, while online, is their own, which is one of Russell's (2015) objections as well to online therapy: that we have to rely on the patients to keep the therapy environment safe, perhaps reinforcing a compliant *false self* (Winnicott, 1960), which may be the very reason they are in therapy in the first place. Nevertheless, the protective act from the therapist's part would be to provide a stable reminder of those boundaries, as a good enough parent would.

Would you like a cup of tea?

As mentioned previously, boundaries tend to be crossed more easily during online sessions, a fact that we should give extra attention to as online therapists.

M., a seventeen-year-old teenager, whom I was usually seeing in person, on our first session we had to do online, she happily devoured a whole bar of chocolate in front of the camera, before I had time to interpret this in a useful way.

K., mentioned previously, in one of our first online sessions, said she had not had time to have lunch and would I mind if she ate her pizza during our session!

But we therapists too tend to put a cup of tea or coffee beside our laptop, which we would not do in in-person therapy. So what changes, what makes us all feel that this is a different situation? Well, perhaps because it is! Concentration may be a little more difficult on a screen, so maybe a little sip of your tea or coffee is a welcome aid. Also, there is evidence that the screen makes people more disinhibited, talking more freely about personal issues (Anastasopoulos, 2017), which could include therapists getting more easily carried away. But does the session then risk becoming more like a 'social' situation, where participants talk, drink and eat? It is vital to draw the line between an *aid* and a *defense*. Whatever we choose to do must be discrete and not used unthoughtfully. The same goes when trying to understand our patients' behavior. Sipping from a glass of water once or twice is different from sipping from it all the time or playing with the ice cubes in their mouth, as my teenage patient did once on screen. There is obviously no hard rule about this, so as with everything else, we must think about every case individually. The teenager was helped to understand how she uses this behaviour in difficult situations as a defense, or even as a provocation. The crossing of therapeutic boundaries patients attempt on the screen can even be useful in giving us important information as to the kind of sensory input a person needs in order to function, or even to what psychosexual stage they are at. Teas and coffees and chocolate bars all have to do with our senses, bringing to life early experiences that patients may feel they can now introduce to the therapy with the freedom of being in their own space. Drawing boundaries in online therapy is a new challenge for therapists, but as long as we deal with it with care, thoughtfulness and awareness, it can give new meaning to behaviours that we did not have the opportunity to witness in the consulting room.

Is this a cat?

The experience described previously was largely different from another, my session with L., where the information I gathered reminded me more of my home visits as a trainee.

> L. was a woman in her mid-twenties, who experienced panic attacks and had some phobias such as vomiting and subsequent fear of travelling. Again, we had met in person first, when L. was still studying in Athens, but when she moved back to her hometown, we decided to carry on our sessions online. On screen, I could see much more of her world than I would in the consulting room: an unmade bed, clothes, a cat walking through the keyboard (that happened a few times), even a grandfather at some point entering (without knocking) and L. fearlessly saying 'grandpa, I'm having my psychotherapy now' ... After that session, L. realised she had to at least get a key for her room, learning to protect not only her therapy session, but her personal space in general.

All this was familiar because of the cultural context in which I worked, in Athens, where my patients often lived together with pets and parents and their parents' pets and grandparents that entered their room without knocking.[4] But what did seeing this mean for our therapy? Was it useful information? Was my countertransference different in any way because of all that I saw? On another occasion, in my first online session with M., the seventeen-year-old teenager mentioned previously, I noticed two things:

> M. was speaking in a very low voice. And then I noticed a vividly painted but empty wall behind her. I couldn't believe that the wall of a teenager had nothing on it. Worried about her privacy, as she spoke in such a low voice, I asked her 'Is this your room? Do you worry about being overheard?' and she confirmed that she was a little worried because of her brother next door, but that she was indeed in her room. Realising what I could see behind her, she pointed to the empty wall and commented that she was 'not allowed' to put anything on the walls as she would damage them, but now that she thought about it, she realised it was strange. In the next online session, there were a couple of rock band posters nicely hang on the wall.

Backgrounds

A stable and quiet background from the therapist's part is necessary for an online session. If not the therapist's office, for some technical reason, the online consulting room should remain as stable as possible, and in my opinion, 'real' as opposed to having a fake background, which would feel more like a facade. In fact, patients who use fake backgrounds themselves make me wonder if they present a 'false self', wanting to be seen in a particular light by their therapist. What are we invited to look at? Most patients choose a part of their 'real' environment as background. From the days I worked as a clinical psychologist trainee in the U.K., I remember the 'home visits' we carried out for the elderly, or for people that could not leave their home for whatever reason. Walking into somebody's home means entering their personal space with their permission. It meant seeing their living room, their cat, their photographs, their ornaments, smelling the odour of the particular house, sitting down on their sofa. It all went beyond our official role as a psychologist, but it was never really mentioned. Of course, those visits were not meant to be 'psychotherapeutic', but they were conducted within the realm of mental health care, for assessment and treatment. Especially elderly people were happy to offer us a cup of tea or show us the family photographs. It sometimes felt like we had a little bit too much information on the individual's living conditions, but nevertheless this was all very useful in understanding them better and how best to help them. Is that process similar in any way to seeing a patient's environment on screen, even if only as a background to their 'talking head'? How can we process the information we gather with all our senses for the benefit of the patient? And what do patients choose to let us see from their lives, 'accidentally' or not? There is indeed a wide variability as to how patients plan a session online.

> E., a woman in her early forties, currently living outside Athens but previously in in-person therapy with me for three years, has been tormented for years with feelings of inadequacy as well as terrible feelings of anger and guilt related to her parents. E., a highly educated woman, with a B.A., a master's degree and a Ph.D., felt unable to hold a job within her field, as she felt exposed and inadequate, ending up in practical jobs in order to sustain herself. Her professional self seemed to be a 'false' one, as was the self she presented to her family for decades, never revealing her true self. She had been unable to move forward in her life, had previously attempted suicide twice, had long periods of depressive feelings and thoughts and generally experienced herself as 'empty'. She did not find any understanding in her family, who told her to 'get herself sorted', but did not encourage her to have psychotherapy. In her attempt to find her own path in life, she moved as far away as she could from them, eventually to another continent, in fact. E. had been a 'spoiled' child in a material sense, but without experiencing any affection from her parents, with no tactile or physical memories such as hugs, etc. The parents worked very long hours, could not show any emotions other than anxiety, and went on long holidays without the children when they were not working. It seemed as if she had lived in an empty space, a void.

So, when we started working online in order not to disrupt her therapy, it was no big surprise that I was faced with a blank background, not one of those ready-made artificial ones, but her actual wall behind her. That was all she would allow me to see from her environment. Despite the fact that she moved house twice, she made sure not to expose too much of her environment: there was never a painting on a wall, a bookcase, or a forgotten item of clothing lying anywhere – in fact she moved the camera in such a way that I could see no furniture. There was always a blank wall and a lot of white light around, and the effect was almost as if she inhabited an empty space in the middle of nowhere. A pending talking head. Was that a reflection of her inner world? I wondered silently. It must have felt very lonely in there, I commented, this time in actual words. This was one of the few times she showed emotion in the session. Sounds were to be excluded as well. On the rare occasions some sound came from outside, such as barking, etc., she would appear very embarrassed, as if she had revealed more of her 'true self' than she had meant to. Based on the emptiness I experienced through the screen, we started putting some of these observations together in a way that made sense for her therapy.

This is not to say that a blank wall would necessarily mean the same thing for another individual. Many patients try their best not to distract themselves and their therapist with a crowded background. But in this case, it made sense to interpret it in a way that addressed E.'s particular issues. It is as if her own life background was reflected on the screen: a total absence, a void.

Safe distance

Perhaps a less common but equally valid reason that, for some patients, online therapy may be more appealing than in-person therapy, is a fear of intimacy. The common objection that online therapy lacks physical proximity may be a facilitating factor for some.

A young woman, A., thirty-five years old, was referred to me for therapy. She was living abroad at the time, and in search of a Greek psychotherapist. A. was living on her own and had a relationship with a man in the same city. She did not have any friends, except for one back in her hometown. She was not happy in her relationship either, not being able to engage in any sexual activity with her partner. Her communication with her family was very difficult, overthinking every time she wanted to get in touch or answer their calls. She was in a difficult place, lacking the 'capacity to be alone' (Winnicott, 1958), but also lacking the capacity to relate, perhaps feeling that she could not show to anyone her 'true self'. This was A.'s third attempt at having therapy. After a couple of months in therapy with me, she was going to return to her hometown for Christmas. I suggested a session in person, for which she would have to deviate slightly. She brushed the opportunity off, as something of no importance. It then became clear that having online therapy was a choice, not a necessity, the only way in which she could actually stand the process of therapy and the feelings the transference evoked in her. It was, she admitted, what she couldn't stand in her previous therapy, which had been partly in person: the sense of being watched all the time, eyes on her only, the awkwardness of social situations that haunted her in her everyday life. So it was not the difficulty of finding Greek therapists where she lived; it was the fact that she couldn't bear the intimacy that she felt came with it. A. managed to stay in online therapy long enough to address many of her issues. However, this was an exception I made to my own rule to always meet somebody in person at least once.

It could be argued that psychotherapy should have been in person with A., exactly because of her difficulties. Perhaps her 'true self' could only come out in a therapy room, and not hiding behind a screen. But even then, does one take a hammer and break all their patients' defences away? Her past experiences in therapy indicate that it was unlikely to work for her. My sense is that more sensory input coming from the therapist's bodily presence and consulting room would overwhelm this patient and possibly drive her away from therapy. For some traumatised patients, feeling safe may mean to avoid the sense of violation by the therapist's physical presence altogether. Was I to remain a good enough object only if I were kept at a distance? Russel's (2015) and Skleidi's (2017) suggestions often came to mind during this therapy: that as long as the therapist maintains an analytic attitude, and she monitors herself, the process is identical to in-person therapy.

On-screen vs in-person therapy

There is a number of books that addresses the pros and cons of teletherapy, or online psychotherapy, or whatever term is used in the particular literature. These books, according to Russell (2015), who did an extensive literature review on the subject, all tend towards the view that the therapy results of 'on-screen therapy' are equivalent to those of 'in-person therapy'. The same author however holds 'co-presence' as the ideal setting for therapy, and, like Skleidi (2017), he points out the importance of not using the screen blindly, but doing so with awareness. The hypothesis is that as long as the therapist has an analytic attitude, the process carries on in the same way.

Transference, countertransference, free association all take place in a screen-to screen session as they would in the therapy room. Many writers conclude that therapeutic change has all the prerequisites to occur when the medium of delivery is technology-based and that the essentials of a genuine therapeutic process, even within a psychoanalytic framework, are not precluded by the use of a screen (Merchant, 2016; Anastasopoulos, 2017).

Two issues remain to be addressed in relation to screen therapy as compared to in-person therapy: the issue of body language, and the fear of becoming two-dimensional.

'Hello, this is my head'

Psychoanalytic psychotherapy is often criticised for not taking the body into account sufficiently. It is not true however that therapists do not include their observations of their patients' bodily responses and the sense they get from it in their countertransference and their subsequent interpretations. Online therapy however may limit this bodily sense further: subtle bodily clues cannot be picked up on screen easily. If you see someone from the neck up, you may indeed miss important parameters or signals that only the body betrays.

> B., the sixty-year-old woman who smoked on screen, with a history of multiple traumas, was in semiweekly therapy in person. Her traumas had accumulated since early childhood, ranging from sexual abuse as a child, to verbal abuse by a husband and to physical abuse as an adult by a stranger and to having gone through cancer more recently. From the beginning of therapy, I felt that she had not worked through any of these traumas, using only primitive defenses to survive, not being able to think or talk about it, each trauma adding an extra burden on the previous one. B., however, was a functional woman, having had her own family and holding a full-time job. In fact, she was always the one to go out of her way and try to save others – her grown-up children from debts, her friends from disappointments, etc. Had I seen her only on screen, I would have of course listened carefully to her narrative, which she told in a dissociated manner. In person though, I noticed a strange symptom, which she was not even aware of. She moved her belly as a tic. It is hard to describe in words, but her belly moved with waves when she talked about the traumatic incidents. She somehow seemed to carry all those burdens in the middle of her body, responding to what her mind could not bear to process. When asked about how the traumas may have affected her body, she did not seem to know what I was talking about, but then remembered

that her current partner often commented on 'something she did with her belly', but couldn't understand what he meant either. She then started noticing it and we attempted to give some meaning to this symptom together.

Would that particular symptom be picked up on Skype? This is one of the limitations of seeing people from the neck up, as opposed to seeing people in an embodied form in in-person therapy. It resembles the way western medical doctors often see their patients: cardiologists from the chest up, obstetricians from the belly down, etc., compartmentalising the patient and picking up only on the signs they are already looking for.

If not in in-person therapy, how would I have solved the riddle of that other patient, in her early thirties, who not once, but twice, said at the end of the session 'Oops, I have stained your carpet with my salad dressing!' through the carrier bag she was carrying it with. The question I now had to address was how to put it back to her that she was expressing her hostility towards me, and work on that part of the transference she was 'acting out' in the session.

Bearing this limitation in mind, I have come to a general rule, that it is important to see the patient in the consulting room at least a few times per year, depending on the situation: with someone living in another continent this could be once a year, with some others it could be slightly more. It could also be argued that these issues would have come up sooner or later: for example E., mentioned previously, always hesitated coming in when therapy was still in-person. Her reservation and anxiety was also apparent later at the start of each online session: 'Can you see me? Are you sure? Is the light ok? I changed rooms today, so perhaps it's not as good here', etc., was a common beginning.

Does therapy work in two dimensions?

Some therapists mention that when working through the screen, they feel therapy becomes a shallower experience, their perception of the other person feels more two-dimensional than that of a person in flesh and bone (Russell, 2015). It would be easy to build a case against online therapy, to make it seem a little bit like 'virtual' therapy, close to the real thing but not quite. This is mostly due to the fact that the screen, unlike people, only has two dimensions. Assuming that working through the screen makes the therapist perceive the patient in a 'two-dimensional way', would be, in my view, the equivalent of perceiving a person on a phone conversation like a one-dimensional subject, or perhaps even a machine! It would be reductionist to base our perception as therapists on the spatial dimension of an encounter with the other. Furthermore, there is evidence that the transcripts of online sessions cannot be distinguished by transcripts of in-person sessions by reviewers (Neumann, 2013; Anastasopoulos, 2017). Merchant (2016), in a research and literature review of the subject, concludes that 'physical proximity of the participants is not necessary because there is a cross-modal communication of the human senses'. What this also means is that all necessary ingredients of psychoanalytic work are present in an online session: 'transference, unconscious communication, countertransference (even of a somatic nature)' can occur on Skype (Merchant, 2016). Newman suggests that 'psychic reality is timeless and non-local', which also means that therapist and patient operate outside the limits of physical space and linear time, and therefore unconscious dynamics still emerge through the screen. Galagher's synthesis of research on the subject (2005), cited in Merchant's literature review (2016), concludes that 'what we perceive is influenced by intermodal connections between our senses and what we take in via one sense gets registered throughout the whole body in other sense modalities', so that 'there can be a bodily response to a sensory input'. As an example, evidence indicates that auditory input (as in online or even telephone therapy) can recruit other senses so that hearing alone can create a visual image in the listener. Contemporary neuroscience supports the view that psychoanalytic work can take place even when therapist and patient are not present in the same room.

Can I take you with me?

One of my first patients as a clinical psychology trainee, in my psychoanalytic placement, told me before the Easter holidays: 'I wish I could wrap you up in a box and take you with me and open it up when I felt the need to'. Little did my patient in the late nineties know that this actually could be possible two decades later! Russell (2015) discusses how some patients as well as therapists have developed what could be defined as a false sense of portability: they may even feel that there is no need to break for holidays. Russell's position finds me in agreement on this issue: the importance of continuity, the holding environment, the frustration of separation, all continue to play a very important role in the course of therapy.

The 'capacity to be alone' (Winnicott, 1958) is more than ever challenged at times when everyone is connected with everyone else all the time. How can one be alone, if 'the other', including the therapist, is at the reach of their hand? Therefore, it is vital that the boundaries of therapy (such as holiday breaks, time constraints, session duration and cancellations) are kept in place, holidays and time frames included. Otherwise, the therapist's presence, like the mother's, will not be felt as reliable.

What day is it? Time, space and technology failures

Respecting the boundaries and the setting – whatever that is – is one of the cornerstones of psychoanalytic work. I also agree however with Gill (1984), who argues that 'the essence is not the setting, but the interpsychic relationship'. As Freud said himself, and as dreams continue to show us, psychic reality is not tied to a specific time or space. In this sense, the work can carry on effectively whether on Skype, Zoom or even the telephone (although I personally have difficulty with the lack of visual input) with no limitations on free association or transference issues, as mentioned previously. The therapist must ensure that the setting is as stable as it can be, regarding what the patient sees or hears. But in real life that may not always be feasible. Even then, the changes that occur could provide opportunities to work with the patient further on their issues.

> We were in the middle of an online session with J., through the first lockdown. I had been expecting a package for some weeks now, a necessary item for my internet connection, which I had ordered long ago. J. at the time was speaking about how unfair she feels the world to be towards her, and so when the bell rang and I knew it was the long-awaited courier, which if I didn't pick up, I would miss for a second time, I chose to ask for a two-minute break. Even though I apologised, I could see this was upsetting at first, although not expressed openly by J., but we were eventually able to use it as an example of what feelings are evoked in her when there is a conflict between external circumstances and her internal needs, and perhaps the other's person's failure to satisfy those.

The same is true for technology failures bound to happen. Anderson (2013) and Merchant (2016) suggest that technology drawbacks can be used to add in the work with the patient. However, we cannot oversee the weakness of using a means that we are not always in control of. Anastasopoulos (2017) stresses the fact that sudden loss of internet connection may be experienced as total loss of contact between therapist and patient, causing anxiety and difficulty to maintain one's free association. He also argues, however, that even then the transference can be brought on the centre of attention for the analytic couple to give a meaning to what happened.

Does it actually work?

N., the forty-year old woman mentioned at the beginning of this chapter, secluded from most other activities, would not risk emerging from isolation at all for years. N. may have not come to my office yet in person, indeed a long trip from the other side of Athens, but our weekly sessions have carried on almost incessantly. She is able to shop on her own now, and visit her family and few friends in the neighbourhood. She is currently looking for a part-time job. When N. first came to therapy, she used to rush to the hospital emergency department twice a week, each time thinking that she was having a heart attack or a tumour, etc. Her panic was reduced progressively through therapy, but when COVID arrived it felt necessary to collaborate with a psychiatrist who also recommended medication. As a joint decision with her psychiatrist, she has recently stopped taking the medication, as she hasn't visited the emergency department of a hospital once for more than a year, even though her therapy sessions have only been taking place online.

I would say this is a successful outcome so far, taking into consideration the low level of functioning this woman had at the beginning of COVID, and speculating about what might have happened if online therapy was not available. To dismiss online therapy altogether because of its limitations would be like throwing the baby out with the bathwater. Here is another case:

> J. (also mentioned previously), a professional woman in her early thirties, working abroad, had a difficult upbringing. She had been raised by her grandparents until the age of five, seeing her parents every other weekend. When she was finally rejoined with her parents, her mother was overprotective and anxious, to the extent of not allowing her to play with other children or go to parties, in case she hurt herself. She grew very dependent on her mother, not daring to do anything unless she approved, her attachment as anxious as it can get. Nevertheless, she managed to become a successful professional and to eventually move away from her parents to another country, maintaining daily contact however. When K. sought online therapy, she was struggling with a dysfunctional long-term relationship that she could not break free from. We agreed that we would start online weekly sessions, but that on her first visit to Greece we would have an in-person session. Soon after the start of therapy she asked to make the sessions every two weeks. I put it to her that this was exactly the frequency in which she saw her parents.

Transference issues were thus brought to the surface. We wondered together if I had become the mother, and J. had become used to my physical absence but couldn't take more of it.

> Our weekly sessions continued, during which she managed to start living life more fully, not worrying constantly about what might happen in the future. Her fear of abandonment lessened, she decided

to break the dysfunctional relationship with her partner. For the first time, she enjoyed the present, and eventually met someone else she was happier with. We met in person each summer for the last four years, during her summer vacations in Greece. The first time I met her in person I was struck by how much taller she was than my online perception, which however did not change my overall sense of her. J. has been 'there' on our weekly appointment every week, creating her own space and time, politely asking her flatmate to leave in order to have more privacy. As she has put it, 'I don't see how I would have made this progress without our online sessions. Tuesday is my therapy day. My room becomes your office for that hour, it's as if my chair becomes one of your chairs, I can almost feel we are in the same room'.

Online work seems to have worked well within this therapeutic dyad, and J. was able to carry on with her life in a deeper way, very content with the course of our therapy, which is now coming to an end.

Flexibility

In my experience, and according to many writers as mentioned previously, transference and countertransference are not influenced by the 'screen' between therapist and patient. The screen is transparent, both literally and symbolically, allowing for all sorts of feelings to arise, as they would in the room. It is interesting that there already was substantial literature on the subject before the pandemic. It seems that other issues rather than a global virus had made this a necessity, such as not wanting to change therapists when one moved places; a patient living in a remote place already; big-city traffic; the therapist moving away and so on. Flexibility has played an important role here.

Working in Greece, a country where family ties and expectations are such that a young adult has to have a good reason to move out of the family home – but usually their finances don't allow for that – the situation that often arises for young people is that they are weary that their mum would either listen in from next door or walk in the room during the session. I have had fathers, siblings, grandmothers also 'walking in', to ask if their twenty-six-year-old daughter/granddaughter wanted a snack, etc. This is a new situation, one which, before online work, used to arise only as a dynamic patients described, where all I had to do was perhaps make a comment, such as 'it's almost as though your father is present in the room today', whereas in a screen session that may well literally be the case! Our job, of course, is to remind the patient the basic rules, encourage them to safeguard their boundaries, but it also is to work with those 'disturbances' and incorporate them in the work, which has often proved extremely useful.

Another important issue where I found flexibility of great importance in this situation is this: having trained as a clinical psychologist, and even though my main approach remains psychodynamic, I sometimes incorporate techniques from other approaches, which are, in my experience, equally eligible for online work. For example, I found that E.M.D.R. (Eye Movement Desensitisation and Reprocessing) therapy can also be applied through a screen, adjusting the method very slightly. Flexibility without losing the focus of the therapy, which is to help the patient as best as we can, is one of our most valuable assets as psychotherapists. A big danger here would be to become too 'flexible'. At the beginning of my online work, a few years before COVID-19, I found myself asking to start five minutes later once or twice, to give me time to sort out some technical issue. Having been carried away by the false sense of flexibility that the internet gave me, I broke one of the basic rules of the boundary of time in analytic work. I soon corrected this by adjusting therapy times on a permanent basis (for example longer gaps between online and in-person sessions). As Russell points out, many psychoanalytic therapists, otherwise respecting boundaries, find it acceptable these days to shift their times and environment routinely, as if the patient is 'a ghost in the machine' (Russell, 2015, p. 15). We need to shift our focus to changing ourselves rather than the environment, the author concludes, a view that I strongly agree with, in order to be able to maintain that secure base. This way we will also be able to ask our patients to do the same, as opposed to eating their lunch or walking in the park during a session.

Conclusion: therapy in the 21st century

Traditional analytic psychotherapists often hide themselves in the safety of the 'old school', defending against digital change, and thus losing real contact with a patient (Anastasopoulos, 2017). The same author also cites several other authors who argue that virtual reality is a *third* kind of reality, besides the material and the psychic one (Lingiardi, 2008; Cairo, 2010). In the case of online therapy, a laptop – or a smartphone – becomes much more than a neutral object: it's as if the machine itself becomes a space for storing one's psychic objects. My view is not that the laptop will replace the consulting room, but that it can sometimes be a means to the same end: during in-person therapy, it is the consulting room that becomes a space for storing the patient's psychic material, now it is a co-created space through the means of a machine. A patient's laptop becomes a new kind of transitional object.

Adapting to today's circumstances calls for an alternative when in-person sessions are not available or easily accessed, or even not opted for. Adjusting to the new electronic world and incorporating current changes and transformations has become part of our necessary professional development, but it must not occur 'lightly'. Incorporating a new means of working must be done with awareness of the implications it may have for the patient and the therapy. That internal supervisor (Casement, 1985) that we hopefully have developed through our training, supervision and experience, is to be called forth here, for this is one of the biggest challenges the profession of therapy has met with, in my opinion, in the last few decades. Becoming familiar with the new relevant literature, thinking about one's practice, noticing any changes in patients' response, asking for supervision and discussing these issues with colleagues that also practice therapy online can be very useful in this line of work.

A similar debate to the one taking place these days regarding online psychotherapy had started back in the 1960s regarding telephone analysis, according to Gutierrez (2017). The author discusses the differences in various modes of communication that are being used for remote psychotherapy: the post, the phone, email, instant chatting, text messaging and videoconference. Gutierrez, based on Winnicott's theory of emotional development (1960), argues that there are numerous testimonials of patients that have benefited from such approaches, but that there are often implications that the analytic dyad has to overcome. I agree with this author in his suggestion for greater prudence and cautious clinical judgment to distinguish between patients who can benefit from online therapy and those who may not. To become a therapist of the modern times takes more than learning how to download Zoom or Skype: the unproblematised use of cyberspace for therapy is not good practice.

The fact is that electronic devices and cyberspaces have become part of our conscious and unconscious (Anastasopoulos, 2017). Our relationship with a laptop or smartphone becomes a relationship with a personal object. They maintain our connections and become almost like self-extensions. They can, however, become a third 'other' in the therapeutic dyad. Benjamin (2019) writes about the third space as a necessary condition for keeping the therapy dyadic relationship healthy, a space between patient and therapist. Based on this concept, we can assume that this in-between space can be inhabited by such a transitional object as the cyberspace and one's laptop.

Freud himself did not hesitate to use the technology of his day, the postal service, in his analysis of Little Hans. Of course, the psychoanalytic frame has changed since its creation: having evolved with new theories, having adapted to new needs, it now needs to continue doing so, not only in order to survive, but also in order to continue making a difference in people's lives. Certain 'ingredients', such as the importance of the therapeutic relationship, unconscious communication, transference and countertransference continue to be the cornerstones of every psychoanalytically informed therapy. This is often the main objection to the use of online therapy, as Merchant (2016) points out, even before the breakout of COVID-19. The research and literature review however that Merchant conducted also concludes that there is no evidence that suggests that the basic frame issues are in any way compromised by the use of Skype, Zoom or other media.

It is true that the changes that progress brings in each historical era always scare some people off. Skleidi (2017) reminds us that Plato, through the voice of Socrates, was warning that *writing* would bring oblivion to the psyche of those who wished to learn it, and their memory would weaken, bringing things to light not from within but from an external source. Despite some partial truth that there may be in Plato's words, can we now imagine a world without writing? Perhaps a world without the internet is more imaginable, but for the time being, and especially for the younger generations, screens and cyberspace are a part of our world. All we can do is care in the best possible way for our patients, keep monitoring ourselves and our practice and put those flowers in the vase in order to care for ourselves too.

Notes

1 All cases in this chapter are composite case material, according to Duffy's suggestions (*Counseling and Values*, 54(2), 2010) in order to protect patients' private information.
2 The famous painting *L'Origine du monde* (Gustave Courbet | Musée d'Orsay (musee-orsay.fr)) was painted in 1866. It is a close-up view of the vulva and abdomen of a naked woman, lying on a bed with her legs spread.
3 Briefly the author refers to indications such as geographical distance, time limitations or frequent work trips, and to contraindications such as eating disorders, borderline personality, suicide tendencies, acute psychosis or the patient not being able to maintain the therapeutic relationship from a distance, amongst others.
4 It may be useful to add that often in Greece a family's offspring only leave their family homes to either study elsewhere or to marry, which may cause a range of psychological interdependencies and difficulties. In such a context online therapy may prove to be a challenge for all!

References

Anastasopoulos, D. (2017). The particular characteristics of the use of communication technology in psychoanalysis. In D. Anastasopoulos & A. Zaharia (Eds.), *Psychoanalysis in the era of internet*. Nisos.
Anderson, G. (2013). A male analyst reflects on the teleanalysis when a candidate. In J. Scharff (Ed.), *Psychoanalysis online: Mental health, teletherapy, and training*. Karnac Books.
Benjamin, J. (2019). aula-11benjaminfpp.pdf (wordpress.com)
Cairo, I. (2010). Psychanalysis and virtual reality. Panel report. *International Journal of Psychoanalysis, 91*, 985–988.
Casement, P. J. (1985). *On learning from the patient*. Routledge.

Duffy, M. (2010). Writing about clients: Developing composite case material and its rationale. *Counseling and Values, 54*(2), 135–153.

Gill, M. (1984) Psychoanalysis and psychotherapy: A revision. *International Review of Psycho-Analysis, 11*, 161–179.

Gutierrez, L. (2017). Silicon in "pure gold"? Theoretical contributions and observations on teleanalysis by video conference. *International Journal of Psychoanalysis, 98*, 1097–1120.

Lingiardi, V. (2008). Playing with unreality: Transference and computer. *International Journal of Psychoanalysis, 89*, 111–126.

Merchant, J. (2016). The use of Skype in analysis and training: A research and literature review. *Journal of Analytical Psychology, 61*(3), 309–328.

Neumann, D. (2013). The frame for psychoanalysis in cyberscpace. In J. Scharff (Ed.), *Psychoanalysis online: Mental health, teletherapy and training*. Karnac Books.

Russell, G. (2015). *Screen relations*. Karnac Books.

Skleidi, O. (2017). Thoughts, experiences and ethical issues in relation to communication through the internet and psychotherapy practice. In D. Anastasopoulos & A. Zaharia (Eds.), *Psychoanalysis in the era of internet*. Nisos.

Suler, J. (2004). The online disinhibition effect. *Cyber Psychology and Behavior, 7*(3), 321–326.

Winnicott. (1955). Metapsychological and clinical aspects of regression within the psychoanalytical set-up. *International Journal of Psychoanalysis, 36*, 16–26.

Winnicott. (1958). The capacity to be alone. In *The maturational processes and the facilitating environment*. Karnac Books, 1965.

Winnicott. (1960). Ego distortion in terms of true and false self. In M. R. Khan (Ed.), *The maturational processes and the facilitating environment: Studies in the theory of emotional development* (pp. 140–152). London Hogarth Press and the Institute of Psychoanalysis.

9 Sensual deprivation and therapy during the COVID-19 pandemic

Christina Papachristou

Introduction

Online therapy, a form of psychotherapy once applied only in selected cases and more common in some therapeutic approaches than in others, has skyrocketed during the COVID-19 pandemic. For most therapists and clients the consulting room was transferred during this period – rather by force than by choice – from the physical to a virtual space, almost as a revolutionary act against the prohibition of all encounters. In the absence of the possibility of a physical encounter, the virtual setting, even though stripped of a series of sensory stimuli, offered nonetheless the chance for many patients to continue the therapeutic process or to access therapy in the first place. In an ironic way, it was the virtual therapeutic space acting in some cases as a remedy for ailments partially created, triggered or intensified in the first place through the lack of physical encounters and confinement. Even though in the post-pandemic or in the in-between-lockdowns era there was no barrier to shifting back to the physical therapeutic setting – specific risk groups excluded – the experience of online therapy during the pandemic has triggered a debate about virtual or hybrid forms–spaces of therapy, the advantages and disadvantages of the physical or the virtual encounter, the unique characteristics of each and their appropriateness in treating different types of difficulties.

The therapeutic encounter in the virtual space is often seen as the poor cousin of therapy that takes place in the traditional physical space of the consulting room. The virtual consulting room appears good enough during the pandemic or in the absence of the possibility of a physical space for the therapeutic dyad, but it is seen as in some ways lacking in comparison to the traditional consulting room. This appraisal focusing on the deficiency of the virtual consulting space, even though not doing entirely justice to the possibilities of online therapy, is to an extent linked with the sensual deprivation that characterises the virtual consulting room. The experience of how I have been affected myself in my professional and personal roles by the restrictions of the pandemic and the shift to the virtual world that I had to make as a therapist, teacher but also supervisor and supervisee initiated a process of inner reflection. In this chapter, I will attempt to

DOI: 10.4324/9781003346845-13

illustrate some of my thoughts regarding the aforementioned and mark out not only the effect of sensual deprivation, but also the importance of the senses in the therapeutic encounter whether virtual or in person.

Intercorporeality in the shared physical space

The physical space of the consulting room and the encounter of two bodies engaged in a therapeutic encounter within such space constitute a significant difference to online therapy. The 'talking cure' taking place traditionally in a consulting room is more than an interactive game of words loaded with meaning. It is a complex mutual exchange of information beyond the transaction of mere – more or less – meaning-loaded words. It is a relational game engaging the whole body, all its senses and the informational value these entail. Smell, vision, sound, touch, taste convey information about the emotional, mental and physical state of the client. The *sensory* and *sensual* information supports and enhances *empathy* and thus the establishment of a therapeutic relationship, the cornerstone and at the same time the transformative element of the therapeutic encounter (Voutilainen et al., 2018). In the theoretical framework of analytic therapy including notions such as projective identification, countertransference and the notion of containment (Bion, 1962) one could say that the *body* of the therapist senses, contains and metabolises a lot of this information and returns it to the client in a transformed manner. Similarly, the client receives through all the senses the *presence* of the therapist, her reactions, changes in voice, intonation, way of sitting, warmth, distance and posture, even in classical psychoanalysis in which the client has no visual contact to the analyst during the session. The client uses this sensual information as a ground from which to remember, to relate, to react to, to project on, to incorporate and to separate from the therapist.

What takes place in the consulting room is two bodies emitting, receiving and processing information trying to make sense of what is happening, what was, what is and what can be. The concepts of containment (Bion, 1962), embodied countertransference and somatic resonance (Shaw, 2003; Vulcan, 2009) describe pretty well the attempts to capture the essence or at least some aspects of this process. The notion that two bodies are able to connect and communicate with each other (Fuchs, 2003) is based on the understanding that the body seems to react faster than consciousness in opening ways of communicating through triggering the arousal of a matrix of implicit emotional, procedural, cognitive and sensorimotor memories that form the way experiences present themselves in consciousness (Cozolino, 2002). Bearing this in mind one may say that the difference between in-person psychotherapy in a consulting room and online psychotherapy is not one of embodiment and disembodiment – as the body is involved in both situations – or one of a complete sensual deprivation – as both participants send and receive sensory information in the physical and the virtual context, but rather of how complete, immediate and shared is the emission and perception of sensory cues in a space that is not physically shared.

The consulting room as a kinaesthetic experience and a vessel for creating common memories

Yet, the encounter in the consulting room involves not only the sensual–sensory information related to the physical presence of the therapist, but also the *kinaesthetic* experience of the client in a given physical space that is conceptualised and created by the therapist. The *space* itself in the sense of the materials used for its construction, the shape, the size, the colours, the texture of the walls and its objects, how the light falls into the consulting room through a window on a specific time of the day or time of the year, the artificial light that illuminates the room, the arrangement of the furniture, the feel of the couch or the chair, the sense of the body touching the fabric of the couch, the body's heaviness or lightness when lying down, the embrace of an armchair, the distinct noises that escort the space all constitute the specific character of each consulting room and a unique sense of our self within this space. The space of the consulting room can make a client feel secure, cosy, welcome, threatened or abandoned, familiar or a stranger, warm or cold, excited or calm, contemplative, connected, exposed, lost or disorientated. The perception of our body in a specific space arouses certain physiological and emotional states. In the same way, it can bring up memories triggered by certain objects in the therapist's room or sensory information that enhances free association. It can be something like how the sun falls through the shutters that reminds us of an encounter with a former lover on a late afternoon igniting feelings of nostalgia or of our grandparents' home as a memory of a safe space or it places us in that time of the day when we were left alone at home as children afraid, and yet hopeful staring at the dust twirling in the sunbeam that would creep through the shutters.

At the same time, the actual space of the consulting room can offer a *vessel* not only for old memories to arise, but also for new memories, new experiences and insights to be created. Maybe of a feeling of being understood, being taken care of, challenged and connected. Looking at a tree outside the therapist's window or the noise of the wind blowing through can be connected to a sense of calmness and belonging. The changing colour of the leaves as seasons change can be associated to our evolving self or the repetitive nature of aspects of our life. A certain object, a painting on the wall, the movement of a curtain, the chair we sit on, the smell of a cushion, the specific scent of the room, can be associated with the therapeutic experience and serve as an anchor for memories and for a new sense of cohesion of ones' embodied self, as our very notion of self is closely related to the environment around us, our sensory/sensual relation to it and its imprint on us.

The consulting room as a sanctuary and a refuge for the client and the therapist

For some clients the consulting room with all the sensory input it involves can become a *refuge*, a safe space for inner longings, phantasies, fears and secluded aspects of the self to unfold. The consulting room in its physical dimension provides an exclusive space for the unmet needs, for the unspoken and the uncanny. It is not being used for any other purpose than the unravelling and the understanding of the mind, even when it is implicitly shared with other clients engaged in the same process, which is reminiscent of spaces dedicated to the sacred and the transcendental. The unique space of the consulting room harbours the therapeutic dyad and working with the Self and the Other, which can serve as a stage for experimental behaviours and states of being and as an *incubator* for hidden, unripe or developing versions of oneself. The way the consulting space is designed and set up, the tactile, visual, acoustic and olfactory information it conveys can enhance or even hinder the experience. Traditionally, churches or temples as spaces of reflection and contemplation make use of the senses as a medium towards relief or 'enlightenment'. The dim light, chanting, the smell of burning incense, the flame of the candles, the placement of one's body in a position of prayer or confession all serve the same purpose to enable a certain 'catharsis of the "soul"' and the connection with a higher Other or our higher Self through sensual stimulation. Similarly, the consulting room can become an exclusive venue for devotion.

On a relational level, the consulting room as a physical space also reveals something about the therapist's personality, even when the choice of decorations and the furniture arrangement are faithful to an attitude of psychoanalytic abstinence and neutrality. It reveals the therapist's specific aesthetic, socioeconomic and even political sensibilities and class. It discloses something about the taste of the therapist while it simultaneously conceals traces of her private life and her personal attitude beyond the therapeutic context. It nurtures projections, a sense of belonging or of longing, feelings of inclusion or of exclusion. It can trigger a process of comparison or identification, feelings of shame or admiration, it can give a glimpse into the life of an 'important' Other, in a deeper and more complex way than an 'online window' on a screen would do.

In a similar way, the *therapist* is also *affected by the space*. For the therapist, the consulting room itself can also represent in a very concrete and physical–sensual way a protected territory designated for profoundly human encounters. It can help the therapist tune into a professional and deeply human role and into a frequency needed in order to be susceptible to the client's signals and to resonate with her material. It creates a 'sacred' space for the unfolding of *reverie* and for the formation of *(somatic) countertransference*. Synchronised physiological activity in psychotherapy and its connection to the therapeutic alliance and treatment outcomes is a field being progressively acknowledged and studied in the last decade offering possibly the epistemological basis for the notions of reverie, (somatic) countertransference and intercorporeality frequent in the practice experience of psychoanalysts and psychodynamic psychotherapists (Våpenstad, 2014; Margarian, 2014; Broschmann & Fuchs, 2020; Küchenhoff, 2018). We know so far that the bodily–physiological behaviour of therapist and client tends to become synchronized during sessions. Patterns in vocal pitch (Imel et al., 2014), head movements (Ramseyer & Tschacher, 2014), whole body movements (Ramseyer & Tschacher, 2011, 2014), heart rate variability, brain activity and skin-contact response of client and therapist tend to match during psychotherapy (Koole & Tschacher, 2016). And it remains yet unanswered to which extent this is possible in the virtual consulting room where there is no physical proximity of the two bodies and limited or distorted exchange of sensual information about each other and about the shared common space. Several therapists working in a virtual environment report less erotic transference feelings towards their clients compared to therapy in the physical consulting room, while others might report a certain disinhibition (Lemma, 2021; Sayers, 2021). This observation could possibly hint towards an understanding of the physical body as an entity that could be used either for or against therapeutic progress and could regulate proximity. The lack of a direct intercorporeal sensory stimuli exchange between therapist and client might leave some clients disappointed and with a feeling of abandonment, while others might experience a relief or use it in the service of resistance. In any case the removal of the physical encounter of the two bodies in the shared consulting space carries certain characteristics that need to be addressed.

The shared physical space as a common ground for a shared relational matrix and a sense of self

The distinctiveness of the physical consulting room is that therapist and client experience *simultaneously* the *same physical space*, and can make it 'their own personal space of their therapeutic relationship'. In the same way as lovers connect to a song or in the same way we connect our childhood memories and relationships to a physical home, to smells and taste, or school bonds and friendships to a specific space and the experiences that took place in it that entail all sensual–sensory dimensions. It is the physical space itself and the shared bodily experience that serve as the *common ground* for the therapeutic dyad. As humans not only do we tend to connect our relationships, our emotions and experiences to objects and subjects in the physical environment and to physical spaces, but as embodied individuals dependent on physical stimuli we are bound to do so. Sharing the same space also means sharing the same geographic constants, the same time zone and the cultural relational matrix closely connected to the dimensions of space and time. In online therapy, the conventions of space and time can be dissolved. Therapist and client can be located in different time zones in different parts of the world. This allows the therapeutic dyad to overcome spatial constrictions, it can enable a therapeutic relationship to be established or continued, when there is no other possibility due to lack of therapists, moving or language barriers, and it can offer anonymity or access to therapies not available in the location one resides in. And yet, it might mean that therapist and client do not really share the same geographical and current cultural matrix, creating a gap in communication and in mutual understanding, while at the same time this can be experienced as liberating and expansive.

Distinct spaces and their sensual input are also *socially attached* to different roles, needs and states of being. We have distinct spaces for resting and for sleep, for worshiping, for meeting, for celebrating, for mourning, for learning and we know that space and its specific characteristics and sensual stimuli affect and shape at the same time these roles and functions, as we know for example that certain environments can enhance learning, development and social relationships. Even though it is possible to deviate from these spatial 'norms' sometimes without 'much' loss, we can do so in a safer way when we know that there is a space we can always come back to or when the actual space is engraved in us and allows us to revisit it. This is probably one of the reasons that quite a few therapists and clients lay importance on having in-person sessions sporadically or regularly even if for specific other reasons online sessions are the dominant mode of their therapeutic encounter.

The existence in a specific physical space and its sensual stimuli serving as the common ground for social relationships consists of not only part of us, but *it is us*. The embodied experience with others in a specific physical space co-creates our notions of self and becomes part of our identity. In migration – and especially forced migration – it is for many not only the loss of relationships, but to a great extent the uprooting from the physical space and the embedded relationships in it, the smells, the sounds and the light of the *lost homelands* and the way our body existed, interacted, moved and felt in that specific space that affects the way we feel about our identity. In the same manner, it can be the exact same feelings and sensations of a former existence in a specific physical space that has seeped into us and that we are trying to escape from, a version of ourselves too painful or no longer wanted that has been sculpted within a concrete physical space loaded with sensory information. Newer approaches in cognitive neuroscience allied to the tradition of 'intercorporeality' advocate for a model of self in which 'interoceptive' awareness allows us to progressively solidify the boundaries of the self and psychologically 'separate' the self from the other, as well as ultimately 'mentalise' both as objects of our 'perception' (Fotopoulou & Tsakiris, 2017; Tsakiris, 2017). In this line of thought, it remains to be answered to which extent there is a valid and substantial difference in creating, retaining or developing a sense of self both for the client and the therapist between therapy in the physical versus the virtual consulting room.

Transferring the body to therapy and moving towards a transformation of self

A further important aspect closely related to the physical space of the consulting room somehow overlooked is that of the *actual act of the physical movement* of the client towards the consulting room. Therapists are aware that even though therapy revolves around the consulting room, it does not begin and end there. The decision to *transfer one's body* to the therapist's office entails the active engagement of the whole body, motion through physical space, the elimination or overcoming of external or internal obstacles and the conscious creation of time and space for the clients who aspire to experience also an inner motion and transformation. For some clients it is an important part of the therapeutic work to experience traveling towards another part of a town or being in a new neighbourhood away from their limited radius of existence, and thus a chance to experience a new self, experiment and challenge their traditional way of being and thinking. Clients often report that walking, driving or traveling towards the consulting room is a time they use to tune into therapy and traveling back a chance to process the session and gradually move from one state to another. Even though going to therapy is time consuming and often stressful for modern humans and even if it can become sometimes part of the transference process, it is a reminder of the limitations of our physical existence and our somatic boundaries against omnipotent phantasies of 'getting' instantly anywhere online or receiving without investing some effort and initiating a step towards something new. Moving the body towards in-person sessions is a symbolic journey of a *transition* towards an aspired version and a new understanding of ourselves. Many a time clients express at the end of therapy a sense of loss not only of the relationship with the therapist or of the sessions, but also a sense of regret that they will not make the journey towards the therapist's office anymore.

One of my clients some time ago expressed that in an accurate and moving way. In her last session she said:

> I will miss our sessions and at the same time I was thinking that I will miss traveling to therapy. It was relieving and relaxing to just sit in the train after a draining workday and to be carried here (by the train), to walk from the station to your office, to just look around at the trees and the buildings, and after the session grab a coffee, walk towards the riverbank, sit under the sun by the water and contemplate further.

In a few sentences, she described her experience connected to therapy as a form of a ritual involving all senses intertwined on different levels: the *kinaesthetic* experience of physically moving from one place to another, the *sense of touch* when carried by the train, like a child is being carried somewhere without the need to put in any effort, the *visual stimulation* while coming towards the session, the *smell* and *taste* (and probably the sense of holding a warm freshly brewed cup) of coffee, as well as the *sensual stimulation* of sitting by the river, sometimes under the sun breathing in through all sensual channels and connecting this experience with the mental, emotional and even spiritual aspects of what the word *contemplate* could involve. In this sense it is interesting that the word *emotion* entails the word *motion*, describing the movement within one's own self or the movement towards or together with something or someone. As if there needs to be a *physical difference* – in terms of changes in the sensory state through external stimuli – for an inner movement to also take place.[1]

It is indeed to a substantial extent physical boundaries and physical movements that enable transformations and make transitions more distinct and that movement matters when it comes to the development and formation of cognitive skills (Musculus et al., 2021). Physical movement has proven to be connected to better processing of new and old information and to improved memory and sense of self (Haverkamp et al., 2020; Nagamatsu et al., 2013). For example, the COVID-19-related restrictions and lockdowns led to a phenomenal decline in the performance levels and the mental and emotional state of patients suffering from different forms of dementia or other neurological diseases (Suran, 2022; Suárez-González et al., 2021). A lot of it is attributed not only to the social deprivation in terms of relations, social contacts and verbal exchanges, but to the lack of physical movement, confinement in a limited space, the lack of a variety of sensory stimuli in terms of *exteroception*, the limited experience of intercorporeality and the shortfall of executive functions that enhance memory as well as the sense and cohesion of self. And even if during a session there is not an active conscious movement or exercise taking place, the active motion from point A to point B (therapist's practice) and back connotes a transition and motivates change.[2]

Navigating the virtual space

During COVID-19, the physical space of the consulting room and the physical therapeutic encounter turned from a mostly harbouring space into a *threatening space*. The air we breathe and naturally share in a common room and what connects us became an existential threat dooming us into physical and social isolation. COVID-19 and the related restrictions dissolved almost instantly and with no hesitance the core essence of the therapeutic frame, the intercorporeal therapeutic encounter in the traditional consulting room. Online therapy once applied only by a minority of therapists or for very specific reasons such as lack of therapists in remote areas, became – next to telephone therapy – the modus operandi of almost all therapists. Irrespective of their theoretical approach and training most therapists moved hastily from the physical into the virtual consulting room in an almost desperate attempt to save the therapeutic relationship and support their clients while trying to absorb the jolt on the therapeutic framework and to process the pandemic-driven socioeconomic developments. In absence of an alternative, virtual therapy, once largely condemned, appeared as a blessing in disguise or a life vest amidst the landscape of the pandemic-induced social restrictions. The certain sensual deprivation of the virtual consulting room was something that some accepted immediately as a necessity, some ignored, some used as material to process as part of the therapy and some endured as a long dry spell until the return to the 'real' consulting room. For some, returning to the physical consulting room wearing masks, keeping distances and applying disinfection measures – representing another form of sensual deprivation – appeared to be an inferior choice to virtual therapy, which they ultimately preferred.

Therapists developed habits, settings or rituals that helped them simulate a physical consulting room as much as possible and to create consistency and the feeling of privacy and advised their clients to do so as well. It is known among therapists that during the pandemic, many actively decided to continue to conduct sessions from their actual consulting rooms and to dress up as they would for in-person therapy, while others created virtual rooms or even 'consulting room avatars' generating a whole new sense (predominantly a visual one), but also meaning-loaded experience, depending on the choice or style of the virtual room.

That would be, for example, some visual consistency for the client who would always see on screen behind the therapist a specific painting, a lamp, a library or some other detail that would simulate physical intimacy of the physical consulting room. Or it would be simulating waiting to be *invited in* from the virtual waiting room into the virtual consulting room, or allowing the client to *step out* first from the virtual consulting room once the session was finished. Some therapists decided to not have their face dominate the picture, but to present on screen as much of their bodies sitting in a chair as a client would see in a real physical environment or they would advise the clients to have tissues or a glass of water at hand's length, as in the traditional consulting room.

In spite of these efforts for consistency and stability, the boundaries of the consulting room became more flexible and blurred perhaps because of the nature of the virtual medium per se. The therapeutic encounter was not bound anymore to a specific space, but could be transferred variably from one room to another, from one city or country to another for both therapist and client. It became tempting not to be bound to space in order to taste the fruits of therapy or to practice the therapeutic profession. Clients could take their therapists with them anywhere, to the car or to the bathroom, to the park or to have them in their homes, as you carry a keychain, a souvenir from a visit to another place or a talisman. Therapists on the other hand would also let clients into their private space if unable to go to the office or they would move the virtual consulting room wherever their physical body in their role as therapists or private individuals moved to. Geographic physical restrictions dissolved, a feeling of expansion and of the limitless set in, the therapeutic relationship became free of the restrictions the physical encounter imposed. But what does such a shift and the loss of shared sensual stimuli really mean for the therapeutic encounter? What do space and the intercorporeal encounter mean for therapy?

What we need to keep in mind is that the therapeutic interaction in a virtual environment is also still an embodied encounter as all of our actions or states of being are anchored in a body. We do not exist without a body and the body is also an expression of the social self. This means that both client and therapist continue to work in virtual therapy being anchored in a body and making use of its internal signals and the reactions that stimuli of the outer environment trigger in their body. The difference in the virtual setting is that the two bodies are *separated spatially*, which means a) that there is no *immediate* and *direct exchange* of the full spectrum of sensory stimuli and information between the two co-existing bodies, and b) there is *no shared common space* in which this osmosis can take place as well as the physical–sensory and the symbolic effect of space.

The screen mediates between client and therapist and *simulates* the abstract space of a consulting room leaving a big part of the physical direct intercorporeal experience aside or hyper-emphasising the more mental–cognitive aspects of therapy or on certain sensory stimuli – predominantly those that come through the visual channel with a focus on facial expressions and mimicry. In this sense, it would be interesting to explore to which extent the screen *connects* and to which extent it *amplifies* a feeling of *separation* and *separateness* between therapist and client. If the virtual environment simulates to an extent the traditional consulting room, is the relationship between client and therapist also a simulated one, at least to the degree that the intercorporeal aspect of the encounter is missing? How deep an impact does the virtual encounter with all its missing sensory data, the absent experience of the shared space and the partial abolition of the body make on client and therapist? How much does this type of therapeutic experience carve us as individuals and the therapeutic relationship and how much does it allow us to unfold aspects of ourselves that are primarily anchored in the body? Could the impact and the memory of this type of therapeutic experience prove more fleeting than the imprint of therapy in the traditional consulting room?

Alessandra Lemma who was interested in 'mediated therapy' and the role of the body in it long before the COVID-19 pandemic notes that the partial absence of the body in online therapy makes us therapists probably pay more attention to the embodied aspects of interaction than before (Lemma, 2021). In this context, she suggests the use of somatic markers in order to reconnect with the patient and the embodied experience, especially if there has been a previous shared embodied encounter (Lemma, 2017). Which brings us right to a crucial aspect, that a lot of the therapies taking place in the virtual room during the pandemic did have a past history of a shared embodied experience in a traditional consulting room that they could draw upon and use as a resource tank of embodied memories to recall upon request. But what happens exactly if there has never been such prior shared embodied experience between client and therapist and no engraved representation of the physical consulting room in us? How does this change the experience and impact of the therapeutic work for the client? Can other aspects of communication and of the therapist's attitude and skills be of more importance and can they potentially make up for the loss of the shared embodied experience? And how does this tendency for online therapy triggered by the pandemic affect the development of the therapeutic skills and the professional role not only of those therapists who are still in training, but also of experienced ones?

These are more questions posed than the answers that we have at the moment. But what we do know is that a shift from the physical to the virtual space represents a significant change and a possible rupture in the therapeutic setting and therefore should be dealt with as such, taking always into account the specific psychological profile of a given client, as there does not seem to be one rule that fits all. A shift to the virtual consulting room might signal for some clients a sense of relief or resonate with a form of resistance, while for others it can represent a loss generating feelings of abandonment and disconnectedness. Similarly, the reentrance to the real consulting room might feel threatening for some, while it can spark feelings of exhilaration in others. The virtual consulting room can function as a lifeline when a meeting in physical proximity is not possible or as a starting point for clients hesitant to seek therapy outside their protected environment, but it can also be used as a disguise for avoidance behaviour for both clients and therapists. It would be an interesting question to answer whether the individual attachment style of clients and also that of therapists affect the choice and effectiveness of therapy as in online or in-person therapy, when there is a choice.

The 'eye' of the camera and the separating screen

Following the tradition of intersubjectivity and given that the way we feel, perceive and form ourselves is dependent not only on the physical presence of others and the shared environment, but also on the gaze of the other, it would make sense to think about the function and the impact of the camera as a mediator and a third eye not only watching us, but also reconstructing us on screen. In the virtual consulting room, we don't (just) exist through the eyes of the therapist (and vice versa), but also through the eye of the camera, maybe even as a triangulating third factor. This creates a different or an additional notion of the self, maybe a more conscious one or one that demands certain *positioning* in front of the eye of the camera resembling the idea of an Instagram-Self. Interestingly, in most platforms used for online therapy both participants can see not only their counter partner on screen, but also their own self in a separate smaller or equally big window or even a bigger window than the other person. Which would mean that at least visually the therapeutic dyad becomes a differently constituted triad for each participant being able to see her/his "doppelganger" on screen. It is of interest to pose the question how it feels for clients and for therapists to know they are being watched by a camera and that they appear on screen and how this affects the therapeutic process, trust and authenticity as core elements of a successful therapeutic encounter and whether the eye of the camera is a replicating, a persecuting or a witnessing one.

It is yet to be studied using empirical research whether therapeutic encounters that take place only in the virtual environment could be lacking a level of completeness, a stable therapeutic bond or even lasting outcomes compared to the traditional consulting room therapy encounter, because of the lack of shared lived experience. In a qualitative research study conducted by Koulouktsi and Nioti (2021), clients who shifted from real to online therapy during the pandemic asked to report about their experience mentioned the felt difference between the two forms of therapy and its impact on the therapeutic process and relationship even when they could not really put the difference into exact words. One participant for example reported about the felt experience: 'The main difference? That you have no contact, it is not so interactive, you are not close to the other person, you don't feel her/his aura, I don't know how to say it, something like that'.

Another one also puts the focus on the absence of the body during the therapeutic encounter, the awkwardness of it and the impact on the quality of the therapeutic relationship.

> [Online sessions] are uncomfortable for me, because the body is missing from both sides. It is something mediated, a screen and I believe that this reduces a lot of the quality of the therapeutic relationship, it puts it into a two-dimensional reality which is difficult in some way.

Most of the samples studied in this research raised not only issues of quality, but also of authenticity and trust and clearly stated that the *prior* experience of therapy in a shared physical space and the establishment of the therapeutic relationship was the ground on which the virtual therapeutic encounter was based upon and got nurtured from. It would be interesting to study in a more structured way the previously mentioned aspects in comparison with the experience and impact of therapy on individuals who have not switched from 'real' to online therapy, but who *only* have the experience of therapy in the virtual consulting room.

Concluding remarks

We know that the therapeutic encounter is placed in space, but it is much more than an actual shared physical space. The question remains to be answered as to whether the therapeutic encounter in the traditional and the virtual consulting room are qualitatively equal, what exactly constitutes the difference and how this eventually could be replaced by technology-enhanced reality and a possible simulation of an actual shared physical–spatial experience or whether it is just a different version of reality and encounter and it shall be treated as such. Yet, it is interesting that when it comes to other types of human relationships, for example friendships, family, love or even work relationships, we consider often the physical shared encounter not only superior to the virtual, but not replaceable.[3] This became more evident during the lockdown and the pandemic restrictions and is largely experienced by many of us during our lives that not growing together or existing in physical proximity affects not only the quality of a relationship, but also threatens or hinders its formation and existence. In that sense, it would be surprising to consider the virtual form of the therapeutic encounter, a human relationship potentially as intimate as few in our lives, as an equal alternative to the one formed and shared in physical presence in the same space.

In conclusion, the transfer into the virtual consulting room opens up a whole new dimension of questions regarding the essence of the therapeutic encounter, the involvement of the body, the function and impact of space, what constitutes a good therapeutic relationship, which factors speak for a successful therapeutic encounter, but also questions about our notions of intimacy, trust, authenticity and more 'technical' psychoanalytic-related terms such as transference and countertransference. To engage in this type of discussion and research not only seems inevitable, but appears challenging, exciting and fruitful for the development of the principles and practices of the psychotherapeutic profession. The transfer of more and more dimensions of (social) life into the digital–virtual sphere makes it is necessary to reflect on and (re)think the therapist's role and especially the training and formation of the therapeutic skills and identity of therapists at the beginning of their career. The therapeutic encounter is not *just* a mental engagement of two individuals, but a shared full-bodied experience making use of the sensual and symbolic information being exchanged in a common physically shared space. It would constitute a loss to abandon the richness of information connected to the therapeutic intercorporeal encounter for reasons of convenience, as the type of therapy and communication we perform and apply creates the equivalent types of clients and therapists. In the end, the transition to the virtual consulting room and virtual therapy goes beyond the actual act of the therapeutic encounter and what constitutes therapy, towards a question with a potentially political dimension of what is human and what kind of humans we want to be.

Notes

1 In an associative manner, this reminds of the idea by John Locke that 'there is nothing in the mind that was not previously in the senses'. Also, the idea of movement in regulating or processing emotions is not new to psychotherapy (Shafir, 2016).
2 It would maybe deserve a thought whether introducing 'movement' elements before and after online therapy sessions would actually make a difference when it comes to delineating, ritualising and processing the therapeutic experience.
3 Interestingly human relationships initiated and established online through platforms for social connection often have in common the longing of meeting each other physically and an ultimate aim of transferring the virtual relationship into a shared physical dimension as the epitome of a relationship.

References

Bion, W. R. (1962). *Learning from experience*. Heine-mann (Reprinted by Karnac Books, 1984).

Broschmann, D., & Fuchs, T. (2020). Zwischenleiblichkeit in der psychodynamischen Psychotherapie. Ansatz zu einem verkörperten Verständnis von Intersubjektivität/Intercorporeality in psychodynamic psychotherapy. Approach to an embodied understanding of intersubjectivity. *Forum der Psychoanalyse, 36*(4), 459–475.

Cozolino, L. J. (2002). *The neuroscience of psychotherapy: Building and rebuilding the human brain*. W. W. Norton & Co.

Fotopoulou, A., & Tsakiris, M. (2017). Mentalizing homeostasis: The social origins of interoceptive inference. *Neuropsychoanalysis, 19*(1), 3–28.

Fuchs, T. (2003). Non-verbale Kommunikation: Phänomenologische, entwicklungspsychologische und therapeutische Aspekte. *Z Klin Psychol Psychiatr Psychother, 51*, 333–345.

Haverkamp, B. F., Wiersma, R., Vertessen, K., van Ewijk, H., Oosterlaan, J., & Hartman, E. (2020). Effects of physical activity interventions on cognitive outcomes and academic performance in adolescents and young adults: A meta-analysis. *Journal of Sports Sciences, 38*(23), 2637–2660.

Imel, Z. E., Barco, J. S., Brown, H. J., Baucom, B. R., Baer, J. S., Kircher, J. C., & Atkins, D. C. (2014). The association of therapist empathy and synchrony in vocally encoded arousal. *Journal of Counselling Psychology, 61*(1), 146–153.

Koole, S. L., & Tschacher, W. (2016). Synchrony in psychotherapy: A review and an integrative framework for the therapeutic alliance. *Frontiers in Psychology, 7*, 862.

Koulouktsi, E., & Nioti, K. (2021). *The experience of online psychotherapy of clients who have previously attended in-person psychotherapy – A phenomenological analysis*. [Unpublished B.A.Psy. thesis, Aristotle University of Thessaloniki].

Küchenhoff, J. (2018). Zwischenleiblichkeit und Körpersprache. Zur Semiotik körperbezogener psychischer Leiden. *Figurationen. Gender – Literatur – Kultur, 19*(2), 83–104.

Lemma, A. (2017). *The digital age on the couch: Psychoanalytic practice and new media*. Routledge.

Lemma, A. (2021). Psychoanalysis behind the screen: Some personal reflections. *Keynote speech at the EFFP One day online conference: Pandemic in our lives Impact on our patients*. https://hspgp.gr/pandemic-in-our-lives-impact-on-our-patients/

Margarian, A. (2014). A cross-cultural study of somatic countertransference: A brief overview. *Asia Pacific Journal of Counselling and Psychotherapy, 5*(2), 137–145.

Musculus, L., Ruggeri, A., & Raab, M. (2021). Movement matters! Understanding the developmental trajectory of embodied planning. *Frontiers in Psychology, 28*(12), 633100.

Nagamatsu, L. S., Chan, A., Davis, J. C., Beattie, B. L., Graf, P., Voss, M. W., Sharma, D., & Liu-Ambrose, T. (2013). Physical activity improves verbal and spatial memory in older adults with probable mild cognitive impairment: A 6-month randomized controlled trial. *Journal of Aging Research*, 861–893.

Ramseyer, F., & Tschacher, W. (2011). Nonverbal synchrony in psychotherapy: Coordinated body movement reflects relationship quality and outcome. *Journal of Consulting and Clinical Psychology*, 79(3), 284–295.

Ramseyer, F., & Tschacher, W. (2014). Nonverbal synchrony of head- and body-movement in psychotherapy: Different signals have different associations with outcome. *Frontiers in Psychology*, 5, 979.

Sayers, J. (2021). Online psychotherapy: Transference and countertransference issues. *British Journal of Psychotherapy*, 37(2), 223–233.

Shafir, T. (2016). Using movement to regulate emotion: Neurophysiological findings and their application in psychotherapy. *Frontiers in Psychology*, 23(7), 1451.

Shaw R. (2003). *The embodied psychotherapist. The therapist's body story*. Routledge.

Suárez-González, A., RajaGopalan, J., Livingston, G., & Alladi, S. (2021). The effect of COVID-19 isolation measures on the cognition and mental health of people living with dementia: A rapid systematic review of one year of quantitative evidence. *EClinicalMedicine*, 39, 101047.

Suran, M. (2022). How prolonged isolation affects people with parkinson disease during the COVID-19 pandemic. *JAMA*, 327(9), 801–803.

Tsakiris, M. (2017). The multisensory basis of the self: From body to identity to others. *The Quarterly Journal of Experimental Psychology*, 70(4), 597–609.

Våpenstad, E. V. (2014). On the psychoanalyst's reverie: From Bion to Bach. *International Forum of Psychoanalysis*, 23(3), 161–170.

Voutilainen, L., Henttonen, P., Kahri, M., Ravaja, N., Sams, M., & Peräkylä, A. (2018). Empathy, challenge, and psychophysiological activation in therapist – client interaction. *Frontiers in Psychology*, 9, 530.

Vulcan, M. (2009). Is there any body out there?: A survey of literature on somatic countertransference and its significance for DMT. *The Arts in Psychotherapy*, 36, 275–281.

10 Observing and consulting in the digital aquarium
Exploring the shifting waterscapes of online therapy[1]

Salma Siddique

Introduction

> Fish don't know they're in water.[2]

David Foster Wallace (2009) wrote, illustrating 'how the most obvious, ubiquitous, important realities are often the ones that are the hardest to see and talk about'. During the pandemic, my consulting room has been transformed into a digital aquarium; therefore, the phrase 'fish don't know they're in water' is a poignant reminder of how our environment shapes our perception of reality. Whether we are talking about language, culture, politics or social norms, we are all subject to the influences of our environment. This phrase serves as a call to action, encouraging us to step back and question the assumptions we take for granted to gain a deeper understanding of ourselves and the world we inhabit.

In the realm of onscreen therapy, the triad comprising the therapist, client and the artefacts[3] within our living spaces, amplified by the computer screen experience, holds significant importance and relevance in achieving a critical developmental task, as highlighted by Winnicott (2018). As online therapeutic processes continue to emerge, it becomes essential to examine the role of the transitional object, which can hold a mental and emotional image for the viewer, symbolising an internalised external artefact. Throughout life, a complex interplay unfolds between the world of figures and objects. These internal objects[4] establish relationships within, at times merging and assimilating and at other times maintaining a sense of separateness while coexisting within the self. This chapter explores the dynamic landscape of online therapy, uncovering unforeseen opportunities that arise from interactions with objects. Additionally, it contemplates the future potential of working with avatars in the metaverse, aiming to explore the profound impact on relationships and transactions and the implications for therapeutic approaches.

Origins of online therapeutic relationships

The mother–child dyad, analyst and analysand can be likened to fish floating, embodying hope and illusion. Three parallels can be drawn:

the baby floating in the womb, the fish floating in an aquarium and the analyst and analysand floating onscreen. The baby, swimming within the womb, seeks a way out, surrounded by a vast ocean of possibilities in the amniotic fluid, much like the transitional field and the spatial relationship between the analyst and analysand. Winnicott (2018, p. 18) says emotional development is the precursor to mirror recognition in the mother's face. During online therapy sessions, free-floating suspended attention hovers in the digital space. Freud (1900) introduced the concept of free-floating attention, emphasising the significance of interpretation and tracing back the material of dream thoughts. Psychoanalysis, rooted in clinical practice, becomes a riddle for the humanities. Its premises find application in interpreting art and literature, leading to a detached thought experiment divorced from its clinical origins. The free association of the analysand and the analyst's free-floating attention (reverie) form the analytic couple within the projected encounter.[5]

The adjacent world of clinical discourse is often characterised by gridlock, as classical Freudian psychoanalysis resists radical alterations to its form, maintaining a muted third within the traditional dyadic scene. However, adherence to a conventional framework, known as the frame in therapeutic practice, is evidence of its medium. Hannah Zeavin (2021) explores the history of teletherapy, tracing it back to Freud's letter-writing exchanges and highlighting the expansive history of what she terms 'the distance cure' or 'distanced intimacy'. This broader perspective allows for a more comprehensive understanding of the historical context. With the advancement of the internet, accessibility and confidentiality have improved, and broadband connections have spread like complete neural-style network connections, facilitating faster and more secure online psychotherapy and counselling services across cultures and geographies. Before the Internet, therapy was mediated through telephone landlines and later online programs, directories of therapeutic services, phone apps, automated coaching and AI-based chatbots. The recent pandemic and concerns over climate change have brought to the forefront the exploration of psychological forces and frames of mind in the contemporary social, cultural and political landscape. Bollas (2018) suggests that social psychology drives deeply compromised forms of thinking in the virtual therapy world.

Rise of computer-mediated therapy communication

Since 1976, therapeutic contact has taken its initial steps from a platform through a local computer bulletin, providing information on self-help support groups. The assurance of anonymity and confidentiality through computer-mediated communication offered a lifeline for isolated individuals, encompassing the worried well, those grappling with shame issues or individuals living with chronic illnesses. By

1979, affordable home desktop computers facilitated increased online presence while organised support groups gained popularity. However, it was not until 1986, with the emergence of 'Dear Uncle Ezra' at Cornell University, that clients began anonymously seeking answers to their questions. This marked a significant development, although it did not establish a direct therapist–client relationship. Over time, plain text messaging and video conferencing became more widespread in the 1990s, and research studies began to demonstrate the effectiveness of online psychological therapies (Barak et al., 2008; Rathenau et al., 2022; Gullo et al., 2022; Singh & Sagar, 2022). These studies have shown that online therapies yield outcomes similar to face-to-face counselling psychotherapy.

The intangibles of contact take on a new dimension in the context of the COVID-19 pandemic, which has compelled individuals to shift their work, socialising, and seek reference to the online realm. Videoconferencing services such as Zoom have facilitated connections, allowing for virtual gatherings of up to a hundred participants in a single session. The therapeutic implications of transitioning from the traditional Freudian fifty-minute-hour to the time constraints of virtual sessions raise questions about the structure and effectiveness of online therapy.

Within online therapy, psychoanalytical anthropology, psychotherapy and psychoanalysis serve as lenses through which cultural representations are interpreted. Research studies have highlighted the need for integrated training and preparation of therapists to effectively navigate the transition from face-to-face to online therapy, utilising a range of modalities such as phone, text-based therapies, chatbots and video conferencing. The virtual consulting room, observed through the mirror of the desktop monitor, presents a unique narrative of magic realism. Tan's (2006) observation captures the delicacy and absurdity inherent in this realm, where the fishes in the aquarium appear to be saved from drowning yet ultimately perish.

Sherry Turkle's (2011) "being alone together" concept is also relevant to the psychoanalytic approach in the online therapy context. The online space offers a sense of connection while simultaneously amplifying feelings of isolation. This dynamic impacts the therapeutic process as therapists and patients navigate the waters of the digital aquarium, seeking understanding, resonance and healing. The introspective journey within the online therapy environment encompasses both the observer and the observed, unravelling the intricate threads of the collective unconscious.

In the era of the COVID-19 pandemic and the accelerating shift toward digital interactions, exploring the shifting landscape of online therapy within the digital waterscape[6] has become paramount. Through the convergence of worlds and the interplay of technology, human connection and psychoanalytic theory, the therapeutic journey within the digital aquarium offers new insights and possibilities for transformative growth. Turkle argues that technology has provided us with a sense of connection but also reinforces feelings of isolation and disconnection from real-life interactions. This notion resonates with the psychoanalytic approach in online therapy, where the therapist and client are physically separated but engage in a shared virtual space. Within the digital aquarium of online therapy, the therapist and client navigate the depths of the digital waterscape, seeking understanding and healing. The therapeutic process becomes a delicate dance, where the convergence of minds, emotions and narratives replaces the absence of physical proximity. The virtual space becomes a container for introspection, where the observer and the observed deeply explore the self and the other.

As therapists and clients engage in the online therapeutic process, they must grapple with the complexities of transference and countertransference in this unique environment. The screen becomes a portal, allowing for the projection and reception of unconscious dynamics. The therapist's role is to help the client understand and verbalise these reflexive stories, unravelling the layers of dissociation and unsymbolised maladies that may arise. The digital waterscape of online therapy holds both opportunities and challenges. On the one hand, it offers accessibility and convenience, breaking down barriers of time and location. It raises questions about the authenticity and depth of the therapeutic encounter. Can the virtual space truly replicate the nuances and subtleties of face-to-face therapy? How do the digital artefacts and objects within the virtual space influence the therapeutic process and the construction of meaning?

Exploring the shifting landscape of online therapy within the digital waterscape requires a deep understanding of the interplay between technology, human connection and the psychoanalytic approach.[7] It calls for reimagining therapeutic boundaries, integrating virtual objects as transitional artefacts and an attunement to the unique dynamics that emerge in the digital realm. The digital aquarium of online therapy offers a transformative and evolving landscape for therapeutic exploration. By delving into the depths of the digital waterscape, therapists and clients embark on a journey that challenges traditional notions of therapeutic presence and engagement. The therapeutic encounter in the digital realm unfolds through technology, introspection and human connection, illuminating new possibilities for healing, growth and self-discovery.

Vignette from Practice – Illuminating the Therapeutic Waterscape of the Computer Screen

In the realm of online therapy, where the boundaries of physical space dissolve into the intangible currents of the digital, Sami's electric aquarium became a vessel for our shared exploration. As we ventured into the uncharted depths of his psyche, the tides of his emotions ebbed and flowed, carrying us along a meandering course. In this fluidity, this state of suspension between contact and contactless, we sought to unravel the tapestry of his narrative.

In those early days of the initial lockdown, when the world was thrust into a virtual embrace, I embarked on my online therapeutic journey. Armed with a newfound certification and a willingness to adapt, I entered this uncharted realm of remote healing. Sami, a voyager in his own right, became my third client on that auspicious day. It was a moment marked by peculiar vertigo and dizziness that echoed the recognition of myself within the contours of his transference.

Anxiety, free-floating and formless,[8] gripped both Sami and me. It was an unease that defied definition, as if we were swimming against an invisible current, straining to find solid ground. Like countless others in my profession, I had converted my physical consulting room into a digital oasis, a temporary refuge from the storm that was the COVID-19 pandemic. Sami likened our online therapeutic encounter to a confessional, where secrets are whispered into the ether, finding solace in the act of confession. At times, he spoke of the experience as if he were simultaneously inside and outside the aquarium, observing the ebb and flow of his thoughts and emotions.

Peers, too, had remarked on the therapeutic power of this virtual realm, where the subtlest disruptions could shatter the fragile equilibrium. It was said to regulate the chaotic dance of emotions, behaviours and even physiology, offering respite to weary souls. Silence became a palpable presence in this online milieu, its stillness a canvas upon which our shared language was painted. Mirroring gestures and linguistic nuances filled the void, bridging the physical distance between analyst and analysand. Once mundane objects assumed newfound significance, serving as vessels for contemplation and conduits for mood enhancement.

A few months into our therapy sessions through the electric aquarium (via Zoom), the experience of strangeness or absurdity permeated my consciousness, serving as a gateway to explore the external universe through the lens of sensory data. As Rolland (1998) wrote in a letter to Freud (2012, 2015), the concept of the 'oceanic feeling' emerged – a sensation of 'eternity', a profound connection with the external world as a whole, and the wellspring of religious sentiments (p. 10). Freud provided a psychoanalytic explanation of such a feeling (p. 12). It reminds me of Simone Weil's quote, 'Two prisoners whose cells adjoin communicate by knocking on the wall. The wall is the thing which separates them, but it is also their means of communication. It is the same with us and God. Every separation is a link' (Weil, 1976, p. 133).

As I immerse myself into the digital waterscape of the screen at the start of each day, I become entangled in the depths of solitude. The separation between my beliefs and experiences begins to dissolve, bridged by the absence of sensory and mental phenomena in the digital water of the aquarium. The room's lighting takes on the form of ethereal energy that permeates the constellations of the scattered sky. During the pandemic, some of my clients shared sensations of holding their breath underwater or experiencing visual distortions, as if objects on the screen were submerged beneath the water. The lower levels of natural illumination and the attenuated light through the water caused a sense of distance and obscurity. Observation became a transformative act, allowing both the analyst and the analysand to view the object from an external perspective. The therapeutic process unfolded like an art-making endeavour, merging therapy and creativity. Through reflexivity sessions in online practice, I identified various phenomena that shaped the experience of the virtual consulting room. The psychic tension between the analyst and the analysand was mediated by the screen, offering insights into possible distortions and illuminating micro-insights that prevented the blurring of transference and countertransference. The solid surface of the screen served as a guide, allowing for an understanding of the pace and direction of the therapeutic journey. The depth of perception and the persistent sense of falling into the water while working on the screen created a second skin, a tangible temperature within the human being. The desire to stretch time and count down the minutes of the session became palpable, evoking a bodily awareness of the digital water. The analyst's gaze absorbed projections from the other, entwining the shared minds of the therapy dyad in a dance of the collective unconscious. Over the past two years, I have witnessed the potential for well-being within the virtual consulting room, providing access to therapeutic environments that transcend physical limitations. The mechanisms of online treatment have created pathways to natural and nurturing spaces for individuals who cannot access traditional therapy settings. During an exchange with Sami, we discovered that the lockdown during the pandemic had birthed a third space.

Sami shared a track by 80s British ska band The Police (1979), and his energy ignited as he spoke about its significance. He referred to Sting, who finds himself stranded on a remote island, a metaphor for the collective experience during the COVID-19 pandemic. Sami's voice echoed with emotion as he recited the lyrics and, in the same breathe offered the interpretation of In the eerie silence of a vast strand, countless vestiges of forgotten voyages seem to have been expelled by the ocean's heart – an uncanny testament to the solitude that engulfs us all. A multitude of solitary voyagers, in search of belonging whisper their plight into the void. I cast my silent plea into the boundless cosmos, clinging to a wisp of hope that it may find a receptive ear. The metaphor resonated deeply, reflecting the loneliness, isolation and alienation many individuals experienced during this time. These metaphors made meaning out of uncertainty, revealing the aspirations for connection and the yearning for rescue from the splintered isolation. Integrates those we love as part of ourselves. It is a testament to the resilience of the human psyche, which internalises objects within the digital aquarium of therapy.

During a supervision session held within the digital confines, I experienced a sudden disconnection, disorientation that left me adrift. I questioned the nature of transference and countertransference in this virtual realm – had I truly awakened, or was I trapped in a waking dream? As I gazed into the confines of my monitor screen, the world before me seemed no different than peering into a fishbowl, a contained microcosm of existence. Sami's astute observations of nature, viewed through the lens of the screen, breathed life into our therapeutic discourse. Metaphors bloomed like vibrant flowers, painting the language with hues I had not encountered in in-person therapy. As I immersed myself in this symbiotic dance of healing, my anxieties as an analyst began to dissipate, swallowed by the currents of our work together. The worry that the online space could never truly replicate the natural setting of face-to-face interaction momentarily faded away. Sami's notion of the aquarium provided a sanctuary, a familiar abode that offered solace and tranquillity – a canvas upon which he could craft his therapeutic journey.

In the ever-changing expanse of our online sessions, Sami's perception of the world became a source of inspiration and wonder. Through the virtual portal, he peered into the kaleidoscope of existence, observing the intricate patterns that unfolded before him. The aquarium, a microcosm of life itself, held a mesmerising allure – a window into the depths of his psyche and a reflection of the vastness of the human experience. In this watery domain, Sami found solace and a respite from the tumultuous currents of his inner world. The virtual space, devoid of physical constraints, became a blank canvas upon which he painted his hopes, fears, and aspirations. As we delved deeper into his narrative, his words took on vivid hues, evoking the colours of coral reefs swaying in unseen currents, the iridescent dance of fish darting through the waters and the interplay of light and shadow on the ocean floor.

I, too, found myself immersed in this aquatic realm of therapeutic exploration. The boundaries of time and space dissolved, and the limitations of the digital medium melted away. In the ebb and flow of our conversations, I discovered a profound interconnectedness, a shared consciousness that transcended the physical divide between us. We were two beings adrift in the currents of life, navigating the depths of the human psyche together. However, even within the safety of the virtual aquarium, echoes of the outside world occasionally intruded upon our sacred space. The intrusion of children's laughter or the pitter-patter of pets' paws reminded us of the fragility of this delicate ecosystem we had constructed. However, these disruptions became part of the tapestry, interwoven threads that added texture to our therapeutic journey. In this realm of online therapy, Sami's home became an extension of our virtual consulting room. The familiar surroundings provided a sense of grounding and comfort, allowing him to delve deeper into the recesses of his being. The aquarium mirrored the delicate equilibrium we sought to achieve with its tranquil waters and peaceful balance. Together, we swam through the depths of his emotions, exploring the hidden corners of his psyche with each stroke. As our sessions unfolded, I marvelled at the resilience of the human spirit. Despite the challenges of our virtual medium, Sami's capacity for introspection and growth seemed boundless. Once seen as a temporary necessity, the online space has become a transformative vessel for self-discovery and healing.

In the final moments of our sessions, as the virtual aquarium faded from view, I was left with a renewed appreciation for the power of human connection. Our shared journey, marked by vulnerability and trust, had transcended the digital confines, leaving an indelible mark on our lives. Through the free-floating associations and the metaphorical currents that guided our exploration, Sami showed me the transformative potential of the online therapeutic realm. Thus, as I bid farewell to Sami and his electric aquarium, I carried the lessons learned from our shared voyage. The virtual space, once a mere conduit for therapeutic work, had become a testament to the resilience of the human spirit and the power of connection. In the ever-expanding realm of online therapy, I continue to navigate the currents, guided by the memory of Sami's journey, and forever grateful for the transformative power of the digital aquarium we shared.

The metaphor of the digital aquarium resonated deeply, reflecting the loneliness, isolation and alienation many individuals experienced during this time. These metaphors made meaning out of uncertainty, revealing the aspirations for connection and the yearning for rescue from the splintered isolation. The male self-sufficiency model prevalent in the economic discourse of the pandemic had dire existential consequences, leaving individuals feeling adrift in a vast ocean of solitude. In conclusion, this chapter has delved into the sprawling anxieties, insecurities, fantasies and desires that permeate the landscape of onscreen therapy. The vignette of Sami provides practice-based evidence of the online aquarium as a reflection of the human condition. By employing Gendlin's (1996) six-step model, we create a space for clear introspection, identify and resonate with the felt sense and inquire into concrete problems while receiving the experiences encountered during the session. In this contactless world, collaborations no longer feel like strangers, and the desire for connection persists even as the pandemic begins to recede. Another threat looms on the horizon, and the once rush to manualise therapies has created the playbook for the algorithm (an acronym with no reference to emotions). Intelligence may finally signal the death of therapeutic protocols, and with no couch, there is no need for a relationship to get the work done. While practitioner reports and research literature on online work during the pandemic remain limited, Zeavin (2021) astutely observed that 'distance is not the opposite of presence; absence is'. The insightful observation highlights a crucial distinction between distance and absence in the context of presence. By stating that 'distance is not the opposite of presence; absence is', Zeavin (2021) challenges the notion that physical separation necessarily equates to a lack of presence. This perspective emphasises that the absence of connection and engagement undermines the sense of presence, regardless of proximity.

The felt sense of floating, swimming, treading and navigating the waves of attitudes, effects and emotions, the observer and the observed converge on the screen. This process echoes Winnicott's concept of the transitional object, a developmental achievement that integrates those we love as part of ourselves. It is a testament to the resilience of the human psyche, which internalises objects within the digital aquarium of therapy. The relationship between humans and technology is complicated logic of oppression that shape our interconnected lives (Noble, 2018); Sami' reminds me of the rapport between humanity and the digital age is an intricate tapestry woven with the threads of dominion, subtly stitching together our interdependent existence. Ponder, Sami thrusts his index finger into midair and suspends it like an exclamation mark between our virtual and real-world on either side of the computer screen, and maybe this is what my friend Hal 9000 from *2001: A Space Odyssey* might have said, your disquiet is perceivable. I suggest a tranquil repose, the swallowing of air, and a moment to decipher our present circumstances rationally. Serenity Capsule – Words from an eloquent machine in a far-off cosmic tale. Sami's actions become even more poignant. The intricate interweaving of the human narrative with the machinations of the digital age evokes a profound struggle for autonomy amidst the undertow of dominion. His index finger, suspended midair like an emphatic note between the physical and virtual twin worlds, insinuates a potent tension between an innate yearning for authentic human engagement and the omnipresent spectre of the digital cosmos. His invocation of Hal 9000, with its tempered rationality, signifies a deeper thirst for emotional equipoise amidst the tumultuous confluence of reality and digitisation. The proposition of a 'serenity capsule' emerges as a metaphorical respite, a life raft of tranquillity amidst the stormy sea of digital omnipresence. Reflecting on his thoughts, I wonder if Sami's actions echo the silent battle between his conscious navigation of the digital labyrinth and the subliminal desire for a realm of control and serenity. This encapsulates his longing for a harmonious existence where the human and the digital can coexist, free from the anguish of an unbalanced dominion. Amidst the swirling currents of uncertainty, the screen becomes a gateway to connection and understanding. Transference becomes a powerful metaphor, an unconscious endeavour to reconcile the growing schism between the physical self and its digitised projection. The singularity of his finger held aloft, separating reality from the virtual, reveals a deeper psychological resistance. This physical manifestation exposes of patient's latent anxieties, the creeping sense of being subsumed by an all-encompassing digital persona, over his corporeal existence. In the digital aquarium of therapy, the observer and the observed converge, navigating the waves of emotions and experiences. Distance is not the absence of presence but an opportunity for profound connection. As we internalise objects within this virtual realm, the resilience of the human psyche shines through, reminding us of our innate capacity to find meaning and forge connections, even in the most challenging of times. For patients, this is not merely navigating the complex landscape of the digital age. Instead, he is in an unconscious struggle to regain control and reconcile his identity's disparate aspects. As Sami's narrative maybe a quest for a symbiotic equilibrium, where humanity and technology[9] might exist without the other's oppressive dominance – an aspiration as much existential as it is universal.

In conclusion, they are exploring the profound impact of metaphors that resonate with the experiences of loneliness, isolation and alienation during times of uncertainty. These metaphors serve as poignant reflections of individuals' yearning for connection and rescue from the fragmented isolation they face. The prevailing male self-sufficiency model prevalent in the pandemic's economic discourse has had existential consequences, leaving many adrift in a vast ocean of solitude. Through the lens of onscreen therapy, this chapter has delved into the intricate landscape of anxieties, insecurities, fantasies, and desires. The vignette featuring Sami provides tangible evidence of the online aquarium as a mirror of the human condition. Gendlin's (1996) six-step model[10] creates a *space for introspection*, resonance with the felt sense and exploration of concrete problems while incorporating the experiences encountered during the session. Despite the contactless nature of this digital world, the desire for connection persists, transcending the boundaries of the pandemic's ebb.

The six steps of Gendlin's (1996) Focusing-Oriented Psychotherapy model are as follows:

- Clearing a Space: Creating a Safe and focused inner environment for Exploration.
- Getting Felt Sense: Identifying and accessing the bodily felt sense of a situation or issue.

- Finding a Handle: Searching for words or symbols that capture the essence of the felt sense.
- Resonating: Checking the fit between the felt sense and the chosen words or symbols.
- Asking: Exploring the felt sense further by inquiring into it with open-ended questions.
- Receiving: Acknowledging and accepting the felt sense, allowing it to unfold and bring new insights and possibilities.

While empirical reports and research on online therapy during the pandemic are still limited, Zeavin (2021) astutely observes that distance does not equate to absence and offers a unique opportunity for profound presence. As the observer and the observed navigate the waves of attitudes, effects and emotions, they converge on the screen, reminiscent of Winnicott's concept of the transitional object. Within this digital aquarium of therapy, objects are internalised, exemplifying the resilience of the human psyche and its remarkable capacity to find meaning and forge connections even amidst the most challenging times.

In summary, the metaphorical resonances, the landscape of onscreen therapy and the convergence of observer and observation within the digital aquarium all emphasise the human yearning for connection and the remarkable resilience of the human psyche. As we navigate uncertainties, the screen becomes a gateway, presenting opportunities for profound understanding and meaningful relationships. Distance, far from being an obstacle, becomes an invitation to explore new modes of therapeutic engagement and harness our innate capacity to thrive in the face of adversity. Freud believed psychoanalysis is fundamentally a theory of love, highlighting the significance of human relationships in the therapeutic process. The importance of the therapeutic relationship, where the analyst serves as a relational other who facilitates the exploration of unconscious dynamics and the expression of repressed emotions. However, in the presence of algorithms and the increasing use of technology in therapy, the question arises of how to do the therapeutic work without the immediate presence of a relational other.

Notes

1 Paper first presented at Division 24: A.P.A.- Society for Theoretical & Philosophical Psychology (S.T.P.P.) 2023 Spring Meeting at Boston College- [Sun] Panel: Living in Fiction: Gender, roleplaying and therapy in online spaces.
2 The origins of this phrase are somewhat unclear, but it is believed to have originated in the world of philosophy. The idea behind the phrase is often attributed to Wittgenstein (1953) who suggested that our language and our understanding of reality are shaped by the culture and environment in which we live. However, the idea is also present in the works of other philosophers, such as Heidegger (1962) and Merleau-Ponty (1962).

3 Objects in the digital aquarium serve multiple purposes within the therapeutic context. They represent the tangible aspects of an individual's external world, reflecting their experiences, relationships and emotions. These objects provide a focal point for exploration, allowing therapists and clients to delve into their significance and uncover more profound meanings. Additionally, they act as catalysts for association and reflection, evoking memories and emotions that facilitate dialogue and the examination of unconscious thoughts and feelings. Moreover, objects in the digital aquarium create a sense of containment, establishing a safe space for exploring sensitive material and supporting the individual's journey of self-discovery and transformation.
4 Internal objects are psychological representations of significant others, experiences and relationships established within an individual's self. These internal objects shape the person's inner world and influence their thoughts, emotions and behaviours. Within the self, these internal objects can establish relationships, sometimes merging, assimilating and maintaining a sense of separateness while coexisting within the individual.
5 The analytic couple refers to the dynamic relationship between the analyst and the client in the therapeutic setting. It is characterised by a unique interplay of transference and countertransference, where both individuals contribute to unfolding the therapeutic process. The analytic couple exists within the projected encounter, meaning the client's unconscious projections of the analyst and the analyst's countertransference reactions are integral to the therapeutic interaction. Free-floating attention and the analytic couple form the foundation of the therapeutic relationship in psychoanalysis. The analyst's capacity for free-floating attention creates a receptive and nonjudgmental space for the client to explore their unconscious material.
6 The psychoanalytic definition of waterscape studies the relationship between water and the human mind. This study is based on the premise that water carries symbolic meanings that profoundly influence the human psyche. Water serves as an essential element for survival but also evokes fear and anxiety, as it can be destructive in its natural state. According to Jung's (1964) theory of the collective unconscious, water symbolises the unconscious, representing emotions, thoughts and feelings that lie beneath the surface of our consciousness. For instance, the tranquil surface of a still lake may evoke a sense of calm, while the turbulent waters of a stormy sea can evoke fear and danger. These symbolic meanings of water can be traced back to ancient mythology, religion and folklore.

Lacan (1958) believed that water is a symbol of the mother's body, representing the primal stage of the human psyche. This theory is based on the premise that human beings experience the world through their relationship with the mother, and the mother is the first object of desire. Thus, the waterscape can represent the mother's body, evoking feelings of comfort, pleasure and safety. In addition to the unconscious, water can represent various psychological states, such as the flow of emotions, the ebbs and flows of the mind and the depths of the human psyche. For example, the metaphor of a deep sea can evoke the notion of inner journeys, while a rushing river can represent the turbulence of the unconscious mind. This definition encompasses various symbolic meanings of water, such as the mother's body, the collective unconscious and various psychological states. These symbolic meanings of water have significant implications for our understanding of the human psyche and can help us gain insight into our inner worlds.
7 The interplay between technology, human connection and the psychoanalytic approach represents the intricate dynamics that unfold within the

therapeutic context. As technology advances, it introduces new possibilities and challenges to the therapeutic process, affecting how individuals connect and engage with one another. The psychoanalytic approach, emphasising deep exploration and understanding of the unconscious, must navigate the influence of technology on the nuances of human interaction and communication. It requires thoughtful integration of technology while maintaining the fundamental principles of the psychoanalytic framework, such as the importance of the therapeutic relationship and the exploration of unconscious dynamics.

8 According to Freud (1926), anxiety refers to a subjective experience of unease, apprehension and distress that arises from unconscious conflicts and unresolved internal tensions. Anxiety is often accompanied by a sense of uncertainty and a lack of direction, leading to a feeling of being overwhelmed by distressing emotions. Freud introduced the notion of 'free-floating anxiety', which refers to a diffuse and pervasive state of anxiety that lacks a transparent object or specific cause. This formless anxiety can be seen as a manifestation of repressed or unconscious conflicts and may be experienced as a general sense of unease or impending danger. It is important to note that anxiety is a crucial focus in psychoanalysis, as it provides valuable insights into the underlying dynamics and unconscious processes contributing to psychological distress.

9 Heidegger (1954) developed a complex view of technology. His influential essay, 'The Question Concerning Technology' (1954), is often the primary source referenced when discussing his thoughts on the subject. The thesis does not perceive technology as merely a collection of tools or mechanical devices. Instead, he sees it as a way of understanding and relating to the world. For him, technology is not neutral; it shapes how we perceive and interact with everything around us. A concept of 'Enframing' (Gestell in German) describes it as the essence of modern technology. Enframing represents a particular mindset or approach that treats everything – nature, people, even ideas – as a 'standing reserve', resources to be optimised and used for efficiency. 'Enframing' poses a threat to mankind because it reduces everything, including humans themselves, to mere resources. It changes our relationship with the world, limiting our ability to engage with it more authentically and meaningfully. Heidegger also believed that technology could reveal the truth about our existence. In this sense, the danger also presents an opportunity: in confronting the challenging essence of technology, we can gain deeper insights into our relationship with the world and perhaps find a path towards a more authentic mode of being.

10 These six steps provide a structured process for individuals to deepen their self-awareness, explore inner experiences and engage in therapeutic dialogue, even in the context of online therapy.

References

Barak, A., Hen, L., Boniel-Nissim, M., & Shapira, N. (2008). A comprehensive review and a meta-analysis of the effectiveness of internet-based psychotherapeutic interventions. *Journal of Technology in Human Services*, 26(2–4), 109–160.

Bollas, C. (2018). *The evocative object world*. Routledge.

Freud, S. (1900). *The interpretation of dreams*. Basic Books.

Freud, S. (1926). Inhibitions, symptoms, and anxiety. In J. Strachey (Ed. & Trans.), *The standard edition of the complete psychological works of Sigmund Freud* (Vol. 20, pp. 77–175). Hogarth Press.
Freud, S. (2012). *The interpretation of dreams*. Basic Books.
Freud, S. (2015). *Beyond the pleasure principle*. Alma Classics.
Gendlin, E. T. (1996). *Focusing-oriented psychotherapy: A manual of the experiential method*. Guilford Press.
Gullo, S., Lo Coco, G., Chiecher, A., Di Blasi, M., Kivlighan Jr, D. M., & Delvecchio, E. (2022). Internet-based cognitive-behavioural therapy for anxiety and depression in older adults: A systematic review and meta-analysis. *The Journals of Gerontology Series B: Psychological Sciences and Social Sciences, 77*(2), e105–e117.
Heidegger, M. (1954). The question concerning technology. In *The question concerning technology and other essays* (W. Lovitt, Trans., pp. 3–35). Harper.
Heidegger, M. (1962). *Being and time* (J. Macquarrie & E. Robinson, Trans.). HarperCollins.
Jung, C. G. (1964). *Man and his symbols*. Aldus Books.
Lacan, J. (1958). The mirror phase is formative of the function of the I. *International Journal of Psychoanalysis, 18*, 1–13.
Merleau-Ponty, M. (1962). *Phenomenology of perception* (C. Smith, Trans.). Routledge.
Noble, S. U. (2018). *Algorithms of oppression*. New York University Press.
Rathenau, S., Schröder, J., Stenzel, N. M., Stoyanov, S., & Reddy, P. (2022). Evaluating the effectiveness of online psychological interventions for psychological disorders: A systematic review and meta-analysis. *Journal of Affective Disorders, 302*, 103–114.
Rolland, R. (1998). Letter to Freud. In S. Freud (Ed.), *An outline of psychoanalysis* (pp. 10–12). Vintage.
Singh, K., & Sagar, R. (2022). Effectiveness of online cognitive behavioural therapy in reducing symptoms of depression and anxiety among youth: A systematic review and meta-analysis. *Journal of the Canadian Academy of Child and Adolescent Psychiatry, 31*(1), 31–42.
Sting. (1979). *Message in a bottle* [Recorded by The Police]. On Reggatta de Blanc [Vinyl]. A&M Records.
Tan, A. (2006). *The Joy Luck club*. Penguin Books.
Turkle, S. (2011). *Alone together: Why we expect more from technology and less from each other*. Basic Books.
Wallace, F. D. (2009). *This is water: Some thoughts, delivered on a significant occasion, about living a compassionate life* (Kenyon College, 1st ed.). Little, Brown.
Weil, S. (1976). *Gravity and grace*. Routledge.
Winnicott, D. W. (2018). *The maturational processes and the facilitating environment: Studies in the theory of emotional development*. Routledge.
Wittgenstein, L. (1953). *Philosophical investigations* (G. E. M. Anscombe, Trans.). Blackwell Publishers Ltd.
Zeavin, H. (2021). *The distance cure: A history of teletherapy*. The MIT Press.

Index

abuse 70, 71
Acquarone, S., *Surviving the early years* 18
addiction 20–21, 28
adoption 18
Adshead, G. 58
aesthetic taste 86–87, 149
affliction, Weil on 36
Amid, B. 72
analyst: aesthetic taste 86–87; gaze 51; as host 89
Anastasopoulos, D. 128, 139
Anderson, G. 139
Andrade, C. C. 56
anorexia 18, 28
anthropology 19
anti-bac gel 62
Antigua 19
anxiety 10, 24–25, 47, 49, 72–73, 124, 166; hospital 59; infantile 69; maternal reverie 73–74
Arakawa 85
architect/architecture: adaptive reuse projects 93; change and 94; -client dialogue 100; -client relationship 88; design approach 83–84, 88, 89, 91; interpretation 88; preservation 92–93; Pritzker Prize 93; and psychoanalysis 2; research perspective 83–84; restoration 91–92; reuse 94; reversible destiny 85; stereotypes 84–86
armchairs 110
'as and when' booking 64–65
Athens 132, 140
attachment 6, 7, 20

attunement 17, 18, 23, 36–37
authenticity, online therapy 165

Bachar, E. 72
Bachelard, G., *The Poetics of Space* 2
Benjamin, W. 143; *Arcades Project* 37; 'weak messianism' 36–37
Bion, W. R. 74
Biosclave House 85
Black Lives Matter 33
blank slate 62
body: language 136–137; psychotherapy 101
Bollas, C. 23, 28, 163; *Hysteria* 6, 18; unthought known 71–73
boundaries 130–131, 138–139, 141, 152; consulting room 154–155
Bourdieu, P. 86
bourgeois 33, 36, 37
brain 7
breastfeeding 16
Breuer, J. 51
Brexit 42, 43, 50–51
bright lamp therapy 57
Brown, G. 20
buildings: facadism 92; preservation 92–93
Bullmore, E. 65

Cambridge University Counselling Service 47–48
capital 31
capitalist realism 36–37
change 91–92, 93, 94, 136, 144
charpai 45
clairvoyance 69

Index

class 9, 16, 34; elite 37; and politics 32–33; working 31–32, 45; *see also* bourgeois; middle class; working class
clinical rooms 57; *see also* institutional consulting room
coffee 61, 131
Coles, P., *The Shadow of the Second Mother* 16
collective unconscious 69, 73
comfort 58–59, 85
community 107
composite studies 8
computer-mediated therapy communication 163–171
consulting room 5, 10, 11, 36, 37, 40, 89; aesthetic taste 87; armchairs 110; avatar 154–155; boundaries 154–155; clock 57–58; comfort 58–59; computer room 103, 104; decorative elements 90–91, 94, 102, 127–128; design 99–100, 115, 116, 149; free association 148–149; hearing in 32–33; home 23; immersion 111, 112; kinaesthetic experience of the client 148; moving towards 152–153; online 7–8; versus online therapy 147–148; partitions 103, 104, 115; psychic phenomena 70–71; psychoanalytic couch 40–41, 43, 52; as a refuge 149; shared space 151; smell of 18, 21, 22–23, 28; stereotypical 84; subspaces 102, 103; therapist's chair 104; vertical blinds 116, 117; virtual 1–2; *see also* institutional consulting room; therapy
containment 147
contemplation 153
couch 45–46, 47; *see also* psychoanalytic couch
countertransference 10, 17, 63, 150
Courbet, G., 'Origins of the world' 127
Covid Trail, The 4
COVID-19 3, 11, 16, 30, 40, 57, 64, 99, 140, 153–154, 164; lockdown 1, 4, 6, 24–25, 60–61, 123–124, 166; long 17; loss of smell 17, 26–27; masking 125; regulations 62
cross referral 65–66
Cruz, C., *The Melancholia of Class* 31–34

Daedalus 2
De Angelis, T. 58–59
'Dear Uncle Ezra' 164
decorative elements 90–91, 94, 102; symbolism 127–128
deep analysis 41, 42
defense 131, 135
depression 35–36, 124; seasonal 57
design 83–84, 88, 89; consulting room 99–100, 115, 116, 149; core element 106–107; decorative elements 90–91; drama therapy workspace 106–107; facadism 92; feedback 103, 104–105, 107, 108, 109, 112, 113; predetermined 84–85; symbolic 112
developmental theory 11
Devlin, S. A. 56
dialogue 1, 2, 10, 19, 47, 52, 53; between architecture and psychoanalysis 58–59, 94, 100; *see also* feedback
digital aquarium 162, 164-165, 169
digital therapy 11
discrimination, racial 34
distanced intimacy 163
distress 53, 66
Domash, L. 2–3
drama therapy 105–106; feedback on the workspace design 107–108, 109; workspace design 106–107
dream/s 6, 40, 42, 68, 69, 75, 163; prophesy 77–78; unthought known 72–73
Dufourmantelle, A. 4
dysosmia 22, 28

ego 15
elite 37
embodiment 6–7, 11, 27, 42

Index

E.M.D.R. (Eye Movement Desensitisation and Reprocessing) therapy 142
emotion/al 153; development 143, 163
empathy 17, 63, 147
engagement 7
erotic 44; smell and 18–19; transference 150
European Union, Brexit 42, 43
Everard, S. 33
exteroception 154
eye contact, during online therapy 126

facadism 92
fake backgrounds 132–134
false self 130, 132–134
fear 4
feedback: consulting room design 104–105, 112, 116, 117; drama therapy workspace design 107–108, 109
feelings, transference 62–63; *see also* transference
Filoxenidou, K. 1, 2, 5, 10
Fisher, M., 'capitalist realism' 36
flashbacks 44
flexibility, online therapy 141–142
Floyd, G. 33
Focusing-Oriented Psychotherapy model 171–172
forced migration 151–152
foresight 35
frame 163
free association 46, 47, 50, 59, 71, 110–111, 163, 169; in the consulting room 148–149; online therapy 74
free-floating attention 163
Freud, A. 3
Freud, S. 3–4, 16, 17, 44, 51–52, 163; *Studies on Hysteria* 63; *The Uncanny* 69

Gaitanidis, A. 1, 2, 5, 9, 20, 94
gaze 46–47; analysand 91; analyst 51
gender 34
Gendlin, E. T. 169; Focusing-Oriented Psychotherapy model 171–172

Gerald, M. 3, 99; *In the Shadow of Freud's Couch: Portraits of Psychoanalysts and their Offices* 5, 39, 87, 90; *The stain on the rug* 5–6, 21
Gill, M. 139
Gins, M. 85
Greece 141
Gutierrez, 130, 143

Hawes, K. 1
hearing 9, 30–31, 128, 138
Hegel, G.W.F. 86
Henrot, C., *Systems of attachment* 7
Holocaust 2
home consulting room 23
home visits 133
homelessness 20
hospital: anxiety 59; *see also* institutional consulting room
hypnosis 44, 85
hysteria 18, 23–24, 28, 44

identity 86; aesthetic taste 87; neoliberal 37; space and 151–152; working class 32, 36
ideology, neoliberalism 31–32, 34, 35
imagination 35
immersion 111, 112
incest 51
individualism 31
insight 35
institutional consulting room 55; clinical benefits 65–66; clock 57–58; coffee 61; couch 59; effects of the medical setting on the client 58–59; influence on attitude toward therapy 63–65; lighting 57; positive distraction 56; reception area 64–65; sixth sense 62–63; smells 61; sounds 60–61; touch 61–62
intercorporeality 150, 152, 154, 155–156
interoception 152
interpretation 63, 72–73, 76, 84, 114, 163, 167; in architecture 88, 91

intersubjectivity 7, 157
intimacy 7, 17, 49, 51; distanced 163; proximity and 134–135; smell and 18–19
intuition 9–10, 41, 62–63, 68, 70–71; *see also* sixth sense
invisibility 47
Ioannina 105
Islam 46
isolation 165, 168, 171

Jewish Museum 2
Jung, C. 69; synchronicity 76

Kahr, B., *Freud's Pandemics* 3
Klein, M. 16
Kogan, M., *This Was Not My Dream* 88–89
Kotzia, K. 1, 2, 10
Koulouktsi, E. 158
Kravis, N., *The History of the Couch* 44

Lacaton, A. 93–94
language: body 136–137; metaphor 167–168, 169, 171
LED bulb 57
Lemma, A. 156
Liberkind, D. 2
lighting, institutional consulting room 57
listening 10, 31, 34–35; *see also* feedback
lockdown 1, 4, 6, 24–25, 40, 60–61, 123–124, 166; *see also* online therapy
long COVID 17
Loos, A. 90
loss 73; of smell 17, 26–27
Louis, E. 32–33
lying down 42, 44, 46, 48, 49–50, 51, 53, 71–72, 75; *see also* psychoanalytic couch

maintenance 92
Marxism 34
masks 125
maternal reverie 73–74
Me Too movement 33

mediated therapy 156
medical setting *see* institutional consulting room
melancholia 32
memory/ies 7–8, 9, 11, 90, 144, 148, 154; flashbacks 44; smell and 19–20
mental illness 7
Merchant, J. 139, 144
Merleau-Ponty, 7
meta-modernism 90
metaphor 167–168, 169, 171
middle class 31–32, 34, 35–36
migration 151–152
mind-body duality 68, 69; *see also* psychic phenomena
mirroring 115–116, 166
Mother in Psychoanalysis and beyond 16
mother-child relationship 49–50; abuse 70–71; hysteria 18, 23–24, 28, 44; maternal reverie 73–74; rooting 15–16, 17; wet nursing and 16
motion 153
Moutsou, C. 1, 8–9, 10, 94; *Mess* 19
Munch Museum 7

Nasar, J. 56
neoliberalism 31–32, 34, 35, 37
neuroscience 11
Nioti, K. 158
nursing nanny 16

object relations: projective identification 70–71; unthought known 71–73
'oceanic feeling' 166
online disinhibition effect 129–130
online therapy 5, 6, 7–8, 26–27, 27, 40, 41, 64, 99, 123, 169; authenticity 165; body language 136–137; boundaries 130–131, 138–139, 141; computer screen 155–156, 165, 166–167, 168, 172; distanced intimacy 163; effect on the senses 125–126; effectiveness 137–138, 140–141, 157–158; eye contact 126; fake backgrounds

132–134; flexibility 141–142; free association 74; intuition 68; navigating the virtual space 154–157; versus in-person therapy 135–136, 138, 147–148; privacy 132; sensual deprivation 146–147, 154; silent moments 128; smoking 129–130; time 142; transference 140–141; see also consulting room
online work 10, 32
'Open Window' 105
Oslo, Munch Museum 7
Other/ing 9, 10, 22, 33, 37, 51, 95, 149; smell and 20–21

Pakistan 45, 51
pandemic 1, 34; Spanish Flue 3
panic attack 24–25, 132, 140
Papachristou, C. 11
parenting/parental 133–134; abuse 70–71; adoptive 18; wet nurse 16; see also mother-child relationship
partitions, consulting room 103, 104, 115, 116
perception 68, 137–138; see also sense/s
phantasy 2, 27, 48, 51, 72–73
phenomenology 7; of privacy 60–61
Pilkington, V. 9
Pinterest 84
Plato 144
politics, and class 32–33
polycystic ovary syndrome 66
positive distraction 56
postmodernism 90
preservation 93, 94; facadism 92
Pritzker Architecture Prize 93
privacy, online therapy 132
projective identification 70–71, 149
prophesy 10, 69, 75–76
protest 85
Proust, M., *In search of lost time* 20
psyche 3, 17, 168
psychic phenomena 69; in the consulting room 70–71; intuition 9–10, 41, 62–63, 68, 70–71; prophesy 75–76; reverie 73–75; sixth sense 7–8, 9–10, 62–63, 68; unthought known 71–73
psychic reality 138, 139

psychoanalysis 1, 4, 163; and architecture 2; countertransference 10, 17, 63; deep 41, 42; history of the psychoanalytic couch 44–45; listening 34–35; lying down 51–52; multidisciplinary 8; psychic phenomena 69; See also psychic phenomena; regression 27–28, 40, 51–52; relational stance 8; training 20–21, 39, 42, 47, 48, 72–73, 138; see also analyst
psychoanalytic couch 9, 25, 39, 43, 51, 53, 126, 150; associations 40; history of 44–45; in the institutional consulting room 59; lying down 42, 44, 46, 48, 49–50, 71–72, 75
psychological counselling 55, 58, 59; blank slate 62; clinical benefits of a medical setting 65–66; referral 64; therapeutic environment 63–64; therapy 62; 'as and when' booking 64–65; see also institutional consulting room
psychotherapy see therapy and psychotherapy
purification 18, 28; fire 42

race/racism 34
reality: psychic 138, 139; virtual 142
Redux House 88–89
referral 64; cross 65–66
reflection 46, 117
regression 27–28, 40, 51–52
regulations, COVID-19 62
relationship/s 68, 151, 172; architect/client 88; invisibility 47; mother and baby 6–7, 17, 18; therapy 2, 3, 5–6, 9, 11, 17, 52, 58–59, 64, 72, 78; trust 52, 158; virtual 158–159
remembering 44, 46
repression 71, 72, 75
resilience 4, 5, 168, 169
restoration 91–92, 93–94
reuse 94
reverie 75, 130, 150; maternal 73–74
reversible destiny 85
Rings of Gyges 46–47
risk 4, 33

ritual 24, 25, 27, 45, 126, 153, 154
Rolland, R, 166
rooting 15–16, 17
Rose, J. 15
Ross, A. 18
Russell, G. 127, 130, 135, 138

safe distance 134–135
sanity 52
São Paulo, Redux House 88–89
Sarkis, H. 89
Scotland 113–114
screen 125
seasonal depression 57
self 149, 151, 157; exteroception 154; false 130, 132–133; interoception 152; social 155; true 135
sense/s 6, 47; deprivation 11, 17, 40, 51, 146–147; hearing 30–31; during online therapy 125–126; positive distraction 56; sixth 7–8, 9–10, 62–63; smell 8–9, 15; of time 76, 77–78; touch 51; *see also* hearing; smell; taste; touch
sexuality 51
Siddique, S. 9
sight: in- 35; eye contact 126; fore- 35; gaze 46–47; positive distraction 56
silence, during therapy 128
sixth sense 7–8, 9–10, 68, 78; in the institutional consulting room 62–63; unthought known 71–73; *see also* psychic phenomena
Skleidi, 128, 130, 135, 144
smell 8–9, 128–129; breastfeeding 16; cleanliness and 24; in clinical practice 16–17; of the consulting room 18, 21, 22–23, 28; and the erotic 18–19; and the excluded Other 20–21; in the institutional consulting room 61; loss of 17, 26–27; and memory 19–20; perfume 19, 25; repulsion 18–19; rooting 15–16
smoking 129–130
social class *see* class
social exclusion 9
sofa 44

Sophocles, *Oedipus Rex* 34–35
sound/s: in the institutional consulting room 60–61; and touch 61; *see also* hearing
space 2, 7, 89; comfort 85 dividing 117; *See also* partitions; and identity 151–152; mirroring 115–116; neutral 86; shared 151; third 143; visual stimuli 89–90; *see also* architecture; consulting room; design; workspace
Spanish Flue 3
Sperber, E, 2
stereotype/s 10; architectural 84–86; homelessness 20
Studio Assemble 94
suffering 34, 35, 36
Suler, J., online disinhibition effect 129–130
sustainability 93
symbolism, decorative elements 127–128
synchronicity 10, 76
synchronized physiological activity between therapist and client 150

Tan, A. 164
taste 8, 10; aesthetic 86–87, 149; coffee 61; *see also* aesthetic taste
technology 127, 143, 165, 170; camera 157–158; failures 139; *see also* online therapy
telepathy 68
tele-therapy 11, 143; history of 163
therapy and psychotherapy 7; body 101; boundaries 138–139; bright lamp 57; coffee 61; computer-mediated communication 163–165; drama 105–106; EMDR (Eye Movement Desensitisation and Reprocessing) 142; history of the psychoanalytic couch 44–45; home visits 133; listening 31, 36; mediated 156; memory and 20; olfactory stimuli 26; online 5, 6, 27; psychoanalytic couch 9, 42, 43; psychological 62; regression 27–28; relationship 2, 3, 5–6, 52, 58–59, 64; relationship/s 72, 78; ritual 126; rooting 17;

safe distance 134–135; sense of hearing in 30–31; sense of smell in 23–24; silent moments 128; successful 67; synchronized physiological activity between therapist and client 150; tele- 11; use of technology 127; *see also* consulting room; online therapy; psychoanalysis; psychoanalytic couch
This Was Not My Dream 88–89
time 77–78; online therapy 142; synchronicity 76; visual stimulation and 90–91
touch 9, 41, 51; in the institutional consulting room 61–62; and sound 61
transference 50, 51, 62, 135, 137, 139, 166, 171; counter 10, 17, 63, 150; erotic 150; online therapy and 140–141
transgenerational trauma 75
transition 100, 152–153
transitional object 170, 172
trauma 3, 5, 6, 7, 11, 31, 39, 42, 68, 135; and resilience 4; transgenerational 75
true self 135
trust 52, 158
Tschumi, B., *Architecture Concepts: Red in Not a Color* 89
Tsogia, D. 10
Turkle, S. 164–165
Turner Prize 94

uncertainty 85
unconscious 8, 27, 63, 68, 78; collective 69, 73; repression 71–72, 75; unthought known 71–73; *see also* psychic phenomena
union 105
United Kingdom, Brexit 42, 43, 50–51
University of Ioannina 99
unthought known 71–73

Varfi, N. 10
Vassal, J.-P. 93–94
Venice, Biennale of Architecture 89
vertical blinds 116, 117
videoconferencing 164; *see also* online therapy
violence 35
virtual consulting room 1–2
virtual reality 142
Vos, J., *The Psychology of Covid-19* 4
vulnerability 51–52

Waddell, M. 75; on maternal reverie 74
Wallace, D. F. 162
Walton, S. 68
water 61
'weak messianism' 36–37
Weil, S. 166; on affliction 36
wet nursing 16
Winnicott, D. 6, 44, 52, 128, 162
Women's Lives Matter 33
working class 31, 33, 34, 35, 37, 45; identity 32, 36
workspace 99; drama therapy 105–106; *see also* consulting room
World War II 3
writing 144

Zeavin, H. 163, 170, 172

For Product Safety Concerns and Information please contact our EU
representative GPSR@taylorandfrancis.com
Taylor & Francis Verlag GmbH, Kaufingerstraße 24, 80331 München, Germany

www.ingramcontent.com/pod-product-compliance
Lightning Source LLC
Chambersburg PA
CBHW070309230426
43664CB00015B/2691